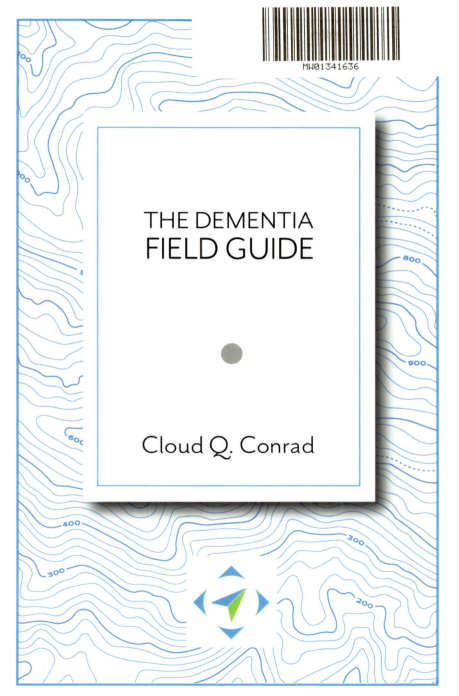

Copyright © 2020 by Cloud Q. Conrad

All rights reserved. No part of this book may be reproduced in any form or by any electronic or mechanical means including information storage and retrieval systems without permission in writing from the author, except by a reviewer, who may quote brief passages in a review. Requests for permission should be directed to cloud@newstreetcompass.com Individual readers making photocopies of the two assessments (Appendix B and Appendix C) *for their own personal use.*

Published and distributed by New Street Compass, Winder, Georgia.

To subscribe to the monthly New Street Compass e-newsletter, visit http://newstreetcompass.com/subscribe

Library of Congress Cataloging-in-Publication Data

Conrad, Cloud Q.

The dementia field guide: navigate the caregiver's journey confidently / Cloud Q. Conrad; foreword by Cloud Q. Conrad

ISBN: 978-1-7358446-1-9 (paperback)

1. Health   2. Self-help techniques

First edition

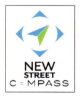

Cover and interior designed by Cloud Q. Conrad
Brain illustrations created by Camille Hayes

MAY THE ROAD RISE
TO MEET YOU —

*In loving memory of James Estes Willingham and
E. Stuart Quarngesser*

ACKNOWLEDGEMENTS

An enormous amount of gratitude is packed in these pages; the contributions of many people are reflected in this text. In researching, writing, and editing *The Dementia Field Guide*, I have been blessed with loyal, earnest supporters who deserve generous and genuine thanks.

First, I feel extremely grateful to Karen Longenecker, Shelley Denton, Becky Tollerson, Peggy Ramsey, Susan Quarngesser, Carson Gleberman, and Mary Ann Willingham. As my draft editors, their unique and diverse input has clearly strengthened the work. Their devoted time, attention, and input increased the value and outcomes *The Dementia Field Guide* can offer dementia caregivers everywhere.

I also thank my public relations specialist, Holly Cline, for her wise insights, encouragement, and expertly crafted book pitches and launch strategy. And to my very talented illustrator, Camille Hayes, I thank you.

I would not have been able to do this without my coach, Shelley Denton, for her inspiring creativity, powerful questions, and steadfast faith.

There is a very special place in my heart for Marie White, Eric White, and Debbie White – my father's home health team in his last year. They each modeled brilliant caregiving, bringing joy and love with every visit. Their support was unwavering. My father adored them. My sisters and I adore them to this day. They showed us the way.

I am eternally blessed with stellar sisters – Susan Quarngesser and Carson Gleberman – my most trusted advisers, most important character models, and dearest friends. Always tight, our sisterly bond was strengthened even further in caring for our father.

And I am forever grateful to my mother, Mary Ann Willingham, for so much love, opportunity, and support through the years. Thank you for believing in the importance of this work. It is an honor to make you proud.

Cloud Q. Conrad
September, 2020

" Science cannot solve the ultimate mystery of nature. And that is because, in the last analysis, we ourselves are a part of the mystery that we are trying to solve."

MAX PLANCK

TABLE OF CONTENTS

Chapter		Page
	Foreword	
1	Dementia: An Overview	6
2	Cognitive Function & the Signals of Decline	16
3	Gauging Cognitive Health	46
4	The Dementia Caregiver Compass	58
5	The Conversation	70
6	Self-Care for Caregivers	84
7	Navigating the Dementia Caregiver's Role	112
8	Why Symptoms Escalate	130
9	The Compass Response Template	142
10	Applying the Compass Response Template	156
11	Resources & Support	194
	ABOUT THE AUTHOR	203
	APPENDICES	205
	APPENDIX A: Wheel of Cognitive Function and Decline	i
	APPENDIX B: Signals of Cognitive Decline Assessment	iii
	APPENDIX C: Caregiver Self-Care and Well-Being Assessment	xv

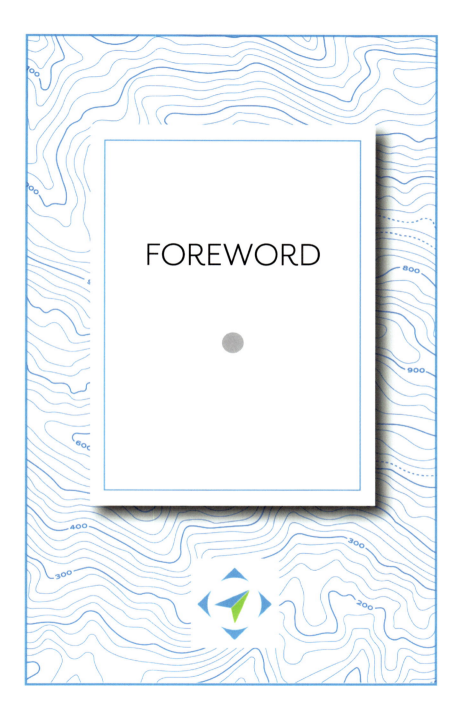

FOREWORD

When my eighty-one year old father fell in 2014, he could no longer continue to deny either his condition or the help of his three children. My sisters and I were finally able to move him out of his apartment and into assisted living, where we knew he needed to be. On my regular visits to see him, I noticed there were many – too many – residents who didn't receive visitors.

It seemed to me that many family members and friends may feel afraid that they won't be able to handle unexpected words or deeds from the person living with dementia, that they won't be able to cope, that the sadness will be unbearable, or that they'll "do it wrong" and the situation will get out of control. So it is all too easy to stay away and avoid these stressful situations.

> *"If he asks me again what time his dentist appointment is, I think I might lose it. Actually, I know I will."*
>
> *"Can you believe it – my own husband accusing me of stealing his wallet?"*
>
> *"I am so embarrassed to take my mom into public places; she says the most inappropriate things to total strangers."*
>
> *"I don't feel like I can visit my brother today. It's just so sad – he doesn't even know my name."*

With education and knowledge of just what is happening to the brain of the person with dementia, caregivers can unlock understanding and create confidence in their ability to engage peacefully and joyfully with that person. And improved engagements make it easier for caregivers, and everyone in the circle of the person with dementia, to spend more time with that person instead of putting distance in between.

If I did it wrong today, I would have another chance to figure it out tomorrow.

FAILURE IS LEARNING.

What I learned was that no matter how "wrong" I did it, both my father and I were better going through his dementia when we were going through it together. What I found was, if I did it wrong today, I would have another chance to figure it out tomorrow. And what I

FOREWORD

know from my experience, my training, and my practice is that the information in this guide is the key.

Like Helen Keller experienced standing at the W – A – T – E – R pump, when she *finally* understood what Annie Sullivan was trying to place in the palm of her hand – letters, words, and the key to a world she couldn't see or hear – you will have the keys to unlock the mysteries of dementia. With these insights you can begin to decode dementia, respond to it, and engage with the person in your care in ways that will reward you both.

It is time consuming and cumbersome to self-educate about the ways dementia changes a person's memory, feelings, and actions. Lots of information is available, yet most sources are incomplete and some conflict with others.

I vowed one day to do something about that. I wanted to help other caregivers understand what is happening to the person in their care, what would change and what would not, how to manage, what to control, and what to let go, without having to do exhaustive research and reconcile conflicting information.

WHAT DO I KNOW?

My father died in 2017, almost exactly three years after the day he fell. After taking some time, I left my 30-year career in marketing and advertising to found a "solo venture" in executive and personal coaching, bringing a good deal of relevant experience forward from my prior life. So I enrolled in an accredited school to work toward coaching certification. I didn't have a specialty in dementia caregiving in mind at first.

That changed when one of my earliest coaching clients, Tara, shared her family dilemma involving a parent's dementia, the denial surrounding that, and the sibling strife and family dissent exposed in the mix. Then, I knew! I would become a dementia caregiver mentor, answering the call I'd heard a few years prior.

Today I conduct educational sessions and workshops in person and online and facilitate two support groups for dementia caregivers. Of course I'll never be able to reach as many people as I

FOREWORD

would like with this business model – there are only so many hours in the day to work with clients in a live exchange.

WHY THIS BOOK?

I have created *The Dementia Field Guide* so that caregivers anywhere might benefit from the methods and processes I use to empower my caregiving clients. It is my hope that you will embrace the principles and practices offered within this self-paced learning format and use your new knowledge to progress steadily to reach a more informed, effective, and desirable state in caregiving.

Imagine a state in caregiving that is free of the stress and anxiety created by using old patterns of thinking and behavior that are no longer useful. This state is filled with understanding and empathy. And this is a state of mind that invites more interaction with, rather than pulling away from, your person living with dementia. This desired state fosters joy and well-being for both of you.

The Dementia Field Guide will equip you with the knowledge, skills, and emotional support necessary to find your way over, around, and through the obstacles that stand between your present state and your desired state – a state where you are competent and confident in caregiving.

This guide is the result of my own curiosity, research, personal experience as caregiver, and as trainer and mentor to other caregivers. Using the foundational building blocks I will help you master, you will have all the tools necessary to identify what your unique situations call for and respond appropriately.

The Dementia Field Guide is designed to be a vital tool on your dementia caregiving journey. It's small enough to fit in your travel kit so you can keep it with you along the way as you navigate the path forward. Until now, caregivers have never had the advantage of a solution like this practical guide to dementia and dementia-specific caregiving. I sincerely hope it helps you reach your destination.

Winder, Georgia 2020

Cloud Q Conrad
Founder, New Street Compass

1

DEMENTIA: AN OVERVIEW

1 | DEMENTIA: AN OVERVIEW

"Is it me?" That's what Martha would like to know.

Lately, she and Jim keep having little misunderstandings, usually about inconsequential stuff. But yesterday was different. They decided they'd both leave work in time to meet at the mall at 4:30, so they could park one car there, and take one car downtown to the recital. Their oldest grandson, James, was performing in his senior recital – the music major's version of a senior thesis – in a jazz trio concert on the state university campus. Each student had only eight tickets to share. Jim and Martha were on his short list.

By 5:00 Jim still hadn't come. At 5:05 Martha gets his text.

"I'm standing in front of the auditorium. Where R U?"

Martha will now have to drive herself, park herself, and walk by herself on the downtown streets to see her grandson perform. She will be late.

Is James' trio first on the program? Will she miss all of it?

Did they not walk away from the dinner table with the same plan in mind last night? Did she make it all up?

Perhaps you've picked up this manual because you're starting to notice some changes in someone close to you, and it's causing you concern. Or maybe it's already clear that dementia is present and you don't know how to cope in certain situations. You may be embarking on a new role as a professional caregiver aiding seniors – many of whom will be experiencing the progression of dementia. Or, you may simply want to learn more about dementia because you come in contact with seniors regularly.

Your curiosity about this topic is real, rational, and should be rewarded. If signals of cognitive decline indeed exist, your understanding about the ways dementia changes a person's thinking, feelings, and actions is in dire need!

We'll explore information for all of these needs in the chapters ahead. First, we should understand the geography and climate of where we'll be travelling.

6

1 | DEMENTIA: AN OVERVIEW

WHAT IS DEMENTIA?

There are scores or even hundreds of types of dementia – with wide variance between multiple authorities' estimates. Alzheimer's is the most common, representing roughly three in four diagnoses of all dementia-related illness.[i]

Many people use the words *dementia* and *memory loss*, or *Alzheimer's* and *memory loss*, synonymously. Memory loss is almost always the first signal of cognitive decline, so it's easy to see why this association is so common.

However, Alzheimer's and dementias of all kinds change the brain across *all* major cognitive functions, as we will learn, not just memory. Thoughts, feelings, actions, and – to varying degrees – personality are also affected. This guide will teach you how dementia manifests its outward symptoms. And you will learn how to engage in ways most likely to promote well-being as the symptoms increase and compound.

Alzheimer's, Frontotemporal (or FTD), Vascular, and Lewy Body Dementias together make up roughly 80 - 90% of all dementias[ii]. Although they share many characteristics, each form has its unique traits. For example, in the case of Frontotemporal Dementia, problems with executive function will appear at an earlier age, often accompanied by changes in personality. Vascular Dementia typically brings visual symptoms such as hallucinations, while Lewy Body Dementia is often marked by motor problems and trembling hands. *Unless otherwise specified, the information in this guide applies to all dementias.*

WHAT CAUSES DEMENTIA?

All seniors will have some memory problems. However, when memory lapses begin to create problems with daily living, or when thinking, emotions and actions are at times atypical for a person, that is not *normal* aging.

Age is the number one risk factor for dementia.[iii]
But everyone ages, so how can we tell the difference between what's expected and what deserves closer attention?

1 | DEMENTIA: AN OVERVIEW

Aging causes changes to our brains that are so gradual they seem imperceptible from day to day. The seemingly glacial pace of even normal cognitive decline recasts the definition of "normal" for that person every waking day. If aware of their own decline, many will compensate in other ways, whether consciously or subconsciously, in order to cope or to cover for their lapses. Therefore it is easy to miss the signals of cognitive decline, and easy to deny the signals we do recognize.

"After all, it's probably just normal aging."

"I misplace my keys, too. So if my sister has a problem because she just can't seem to keep up with her keys, I must also have a problem."

"But yesterday and today, my husband has seemed fine – I must be over-thinking it."

Thank you for having the best caregiving intentions by educating yourself, learning what to expect and how to help the person in your care enjoy maximum health and well-being in every stage of the dementia progression. With *The Dementia Field Guide* you can reach your objective, becoming the outstanding and understanding caregiver you want to be!

HOW COMMON IS DEMENTIA?

Dementia can develop as early as one's forties but more commonly emerges in one's sixties, seventies, or eighties. Our risk of developing dementia increases with age – a phenomenon we all face. Those of Hispanic or African descent are one and a half times and two times more likely, respectively, than Caucasian males to develop dementia[iv]. Two out of every three people with dementia are female.[v]

Dementia affects one in five households today, including the person living with dementia and their primary caregivers. It's a math equation based on the population and number of US households, the number of Americans currently living with dementia, the average number of unpaid caregivers attending to each of them, and the number of caregivers living with the person with dementia.

1 | DEMENTIA: AN OVERVIEW

The statistics used in this calculation are derived from six credible sources including the National Institute of Health (NIH), the US Census, and the Alzheimer's Association. They are cited in full in an article published on the New

Dementia affects one in every five households today.

Street Compass website titled *"Boomer Surge in Dementia".*[vi]

Nearly six million people are living with an Alzheimer's diagnosis in the U.S. today.[vii] (This *does not* include other dementia diagnoses *or* the untold others who are also affected but as yet undiagnosed.) On average, three caregivers (2.8 to be precise[viii]) are involved, two of whom are living with the person in their care. After computing all that math, across the 128+ million households in the US today[ix], one in every five households is affected by dementia.

That's a lot of households touched by dementia. But with the changing demographics of our country and the impact dementia will have on aging baby boomers, who are just approaching the 75+ age bracket today, the footprint of dementia will become much larger.

MORE AND MORE ADULTS WILL BE AFFECTED BY DEMENTIA.

With age being the number one risk factor for dementia, the Alzheimer's Association projects an increased prevalence in diagnosed cases in the coming decades and estimates there will be about 14 million people living with dementia by the year 2050[x].

If the Alzheimer's Association projections are true, diagnosed cases of dementia will almost triple in the next thirty years. On this basis, we can estimate that, including people living with dementia and their caregivers, the number of households navigating dementia is expected to increase to one in two by the year 2034.[xi]

This will mean that, on average, just fourteen years from the date of this printing, *there will be a family navigating dementia in every other house on your street*. It should be stressed that this math is based on projections of *diagnosed* cases of dementia. It is unclear

1 | DEMENTIA: AN OVERVIEW

how many additional families will be affected, but are not counted, in the statistics cited in the New Street Compass article, "Boomer surge in dementia" because there has not been a formal diagnosis.

One in two households will be affected by dementia by 2034.

Having such a profound and growing impact on families and the communities surrounding them, dementia deserves everyone's understanding. Business leaders, faith leaders, civic leaders, and anyone who interacts with seniors in a professional, volunteer or social capacity will be working with, or for, those experiencing dementia. Understanding leads to empathy and healthier, more productive engagement with those facing cognitive decline.

STEPPING INTO THE CAREGIVING ROLE

Let's focus on your household. If you believe that someone in your household may be experiencing cognitive impairment, you will benefit from knowing how to recognize cognitive decline, how to pursue medical advice, and how to prepare for your role as a caregiver. This is often complicated for family members in a relationship that is forever changed and will continue to change.

When the signals of cognitive decline advance to become symptoms of dementia, it will help to know how to navigate through the situations created by those symptoms. This is unfamiliar terrain, and indeed challenging at times. Most caregivers anticipate a daunting road ahead, but that needn't be.

Caregiving is often complicated in a relationship that is changed forever and forever changing.

Instead of fear, frustration, and failure, it's possible that your caregiving journey can be marked by confidence, creative problem solving and competence. Your curiosity can create the difference between these polar opposite courses of travel. It can enable you to land in a place of peace and continued connection with your loved one.

1 | DEMENTIA: AN OVERVIEW

EMBRACING THE INEVITABLE

The brain is a fascinating and profoundly complex system. We can't begin to fathom all the inner workings of a brain in its peak function, or in the forms of cognitive decline that occur naturally as we age.

It is miraculous in the way the various parts of the brain work in concert to synchronously execute simple tasks we take for granted, like blowing our nose, while performing much more sophisticated tasks like preparing a monthly productivity report for our boss. Understanding how our aging brains are expected to change will benefit our ability to adapt effectively over time to each other.

Normal aging slows our cognitive processing. It impairs our eyesight and hearing. It restricts our motion and damages our skin. These changes are nearly universal. But for some, the effects of aging will stretch beyond what is considered normal, thereby challenging daily life.

CAREGIVER APPREHENSION

Given the complexities of the "normal" brain, how could we ever possibly hope to decode the thought processes of a person living with dementia? Never mind being able to respond effectively in the escalated situations commonly created by dementia's symptoms, or steer clear of them in the first place?

Follow this guide and you will learn to do just that. The knowledge accessed here alternates between the awareness I create for you and the awareness that you create for yourself, gained through information shared in this manual, field assignments, skill-building exercises, journal spaces, and assessments.

LEARNING OBJECTIVES

Readers who follow the content and exercises included in *The Dementia Field Guide* will be able to:

- describe eight cognitive functions we use to interpret and respond to our world on a daily basis, and how age normally changes these functions.

- examine the signals of cognitive decline through three useful gauges to help discern whether the changes you've noticed in

1 | DEMENTIA: AN OVERVIEW

yourself or someone else are normal, or cause for concern and further exploration. *A full assessment tool will create greater clarity on the specifics in your situation.*

- discover an orientation to caregiving that, if embraced, will guide your outlook and actions in caregiving and in self-care
- explore your intention in caregiving and define what you'll need in order to deliver on your intentions
- design an action plan to respond to your own needs for health and well-being in the caregiving role
- plan when, where, and how to approach the conversation about cognitive decline
- compose and rehearse your conversation in advance
- recognize common symptoms of dementia's progression based on knowledge of cognitive function and signals of decline
- explain why situational escalations occur
- formulate responses to escalated symptoms that are appropriate and effective for *your* situations to restore calm and security
- interpret the results of a self-assessment for you as a caregiver
- outline the benefits of several recommended resources and support for your consideration and evaluation
- navigate the role of dementia caregiver confidently and competently

I invite you to follow my lead as I help you unlock the mysteries of dementia and chart a course through this unfamiliar terrain. Prior to embarking on our journey we must familiarize ourselves with the topography of cognitive function, detailed in the next chapter.

---

[i] Alzheimer's Association. (*2020). 2020 Alzheimer's Disease Facts and Figures* [Report].
https://www.alz.org/media/Documents/alzheimers-facts-and-figures_1.pdf

[ii] Alzheimer's Association (2020)

[iii] Centers for Disease Control and Prevention. (2019, April 5). *Alzheimer's Disease and Healthy Aging: What is dementia?* US Department of Health and Human Services. https://www.cdc.gov/aging/dementia/index.html

[iv] Alzheimer's Association (2020)

1 | DEMENTIA: AN OVERVIEW

[v] Alzheimer's Association (2020)

[vi] Conrad, C. (2020). Boomer surge in dementia. *New Street Compass.*
https://newstreetcompass.com/2020/06/21/boomer-surge-in-dementia.

[vii] Alzheimer's Association. (*2020*). *2020 Alzheimer's Disease Facts and Figures*
[Report].   https://www.alz.org/media/Documents/alzheimers-facts-and-
figures_l.pdf

[viii] Alzheimer's Association (2020)

[ix] Duffin, E. (2019, November). *Average number of own children under 18 in families
with children in the United States from 1960 to 2019* (STATISTA
https://www.statista.com/statistics/718084/average-number-of-own-children-
per-family/

[x] Duffin (2019)

[xi] Conrad, C. (2020). Boomer surge in dementia. *New Street Compass.*
https://newstreetcompass.com/2020/06/21/boomer-surge-in-dementia.

2

COGNITIVE FUNCTION and the SIGNALS of DECLINE

> While watching television, Andrea feels chilled by the draft in her cabin. She decides to go and get her fleece jacket at the next commercial break. When the first ad comes on, she makes her way up the stairs to the loft bedroom above. But when she reaches the top step, she has to ask out loud, *"What did I come up here for???"* She scans the space. Nothing. After a few seconds, she gives up and goes back down the steps. Hating to accept defeat, she pauses a minute before sitting down. Then comes the tough self-talk. *"I should just admit I have a memory problem."* But as soon as she sits down again, she knows. *"The fleece jacket!"*

Aging changes us. Some changes are nearly universal, like the graying of our hair and the wrinkling of our skin. These changes happen to all of us, but not at the same age or to the same extent.

Aging causes other changes – ones that affect our thinking. It is natural that our thought processes slow as we age. Maybe we take longer to respond in conversation. Maybe we are slower to come up with someone's name if we haven't seen them in a while. Or maybe we forget why we came all the way upstairs, only figure it out when we get all the way back to where we were when we decided to go there in the first place.

Such changes occur because the peak cognitive skills that contribute to social exchanges may peak, plateau and begin to decline in our late 40s and early 50s. These cognitive skills include our ability to understand, follow along and keep up our end of a conversation. Other skills that help us recognize faces and remember what was just said actually begin to decline in our 20s and early 30s.[i] Reductions in peak working memory cause slower response times and "senior moments" every so often – normal aging that happens to all of us.

MORE THAN "NORMAL" AGING?

But maybe what concerns you is a little bit more. Is what you're noticing "normal"? How can you tell if there's a problem that deserves your attention? *In this chapter we will discuss eight cognitive brain functions and spotlight several signals of cognitive impairment associated with each.* This knowledge will prepare you to complete a full assessment of cognitive function of your loved one, which you will be asked to do at the end of this chapter.

THE WHEEL OF COGNITIVE FUNCTION AND DECLINE

For each of the cognitive functions explored in this chapter a summary is included. This information is further summarized in Appendix A: The Wheel of Cognitive Function and Decline. This is a fold-out diagram.

"The Wheel of Function" – or simply, "The Wheel" – captures all functions, skills and signals of decline on one page, arrayed in a series of concentric circles. In the inner circle you will find eight labeled circles, just as below, one for each cognitive function detailed in this chapter. Radiating out from each cognitive function, on "The Wheel" found in Appendix A, are the skills associated with each function and the signals of cognitive decline.

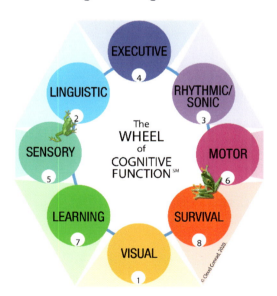

Keep "The Wheel" handy as you review the detailed information provided on each of the eight cognitive functions explored in this chapter. (The image above is a scaled-back version of "The Wheel".)

2 | COGNITIVE FUNCTION and the SIGNALS of DECLINE

The other key visual used in this chapter is based on an illustration series that approximates *Positron Emission Tomography* (or PET) scans for a healthy adult brain, a mildly impaired brain, and a brain in the late stages of dementia.

Basically, a PET scan examines brain activity, based on an image that shows a horizontal "slice" of the brain. In the illustration below, notice the indentations representing the location of the temples, and the flattish edge on top that represents the forehead.

Think of the PET scans like a weather map. The weather map in a newspaper shows the predicted temperatures across the nation. The areas with the hottest temperatures are shaded in red. The next hottest areas are in orange, then yellow, and so on through the color spectrum until we see the coldest areas in deep blue or indigo.

This "heat map" approach is useful when we think about cognitive brain function. The colored shading in our illustrated series describes relative degrees of activity in the brain, with red showing the highest amount of activity, then orange, yellow, green, blue, indigo and violet, which represents the least amount of activity.

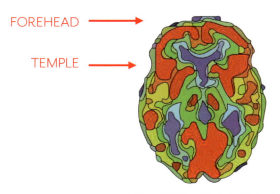

HEALTHY ADULT BRAIN

As we talk about cognitive activity we will compare illustrations of progressive brain scans to comprehend the decline in activity caused by Alzheimer's and other dementias.[ii] Please note that the illustrations only approximate the location of these functions and respective regions of the brain; the illustration presents brain

2 | COGNITIVE FUNCTION and the SIGNALS of DECLINE

activity rather than brain anatomy. Also, we must realize that PET scans render a three dimensional form in cross section – essentially we are viewing a slice of a brain.

1 VISUAL PROCESSING

Place your hand on the back of your head, with your palm cupping the convex part of your scull. This is the occipital lobe. What your eyes take in is processed in this area.

The most powerful sensory information is visual data because, of all sensory information, we rely on visual cues most to process and understand the world around us. Think about it. When you hear a noise, what do you do? You turn around and look. You don't rely on your ears alone. You confirm with your eyes what your ears have told you to be true in order to trust your interpretation of the event.

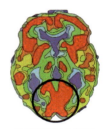

OCCIPITAL LOBE

What *is* visual data? What is it that we *see* when we look at something? The occipital lobe is responsible for detecting motion and distinguishing shapes and forms. It identifies light and differentiates color. It renders dimension and perceives depth.

What we take in with our eyes is sent all the way back to the occipital lobe to be processed into images we can decipher. But, when the occipital lobe is affected by dementia, people can no longer process that same visual data the way they once did.

SIGNALS OF DECLINE

One of the ways decline in the occipital lobe shows up might be loss of object recognition. You might find your husband putting toothpaste on his hairbrush instead of his toothbrush, for example. Or putting his shoes in the freezer instead of the closet.

Similarly, facial recognition can diminish over time. It is normal to have a lapse and forget the name of someone we haven't seen in years. But it could be a signal that the occipital lobe is not functioning normally if problems with facial recognition occur with people seen more frequently.

2 | COGNITIVE FUNCTION and the SIGNALS of DECLINE

Problems with color recognition are another possible dysfunction in the occipital lobe. This can make finding distinct objects in today's monochrome interior color schemes difficult for people with dementia. It may be difficult to find the toilet, for example, if the fixtures, walls, and floors are all white – it won't stand out.

Motion blindness, like not noticing a car turning into your lane ahead of you, or a bicyclist on the road edge, can be another problem and not a normal part of aging. This would make driving dangerous.

Problems with shadows and reflection arise when light and motion are perceived differently than before. Shadow and reflection can create hallucinations – when they are mistaken for strange things or people, it could be a signal of cognitive decline.

And then, there's something else. Hold your arms out to your sides so they are spread at 180 degrees. Now, wave your fingers. If you can't see your fingers, slowly move your hands closer together in front of your body (still at arms' length) until your waving fingers appear at the edge of your vision. It's normal for a 75 year old to have lost roughly 45 degrees on each side, or about 90 total degrees in field of vision[iii]. This **loss in peripheral vision** is not just side to side but in all directions.

Have you ever had to make a pet wear a plastic cone to prevent it from licking a wound or an incision? Your pet has limited visual

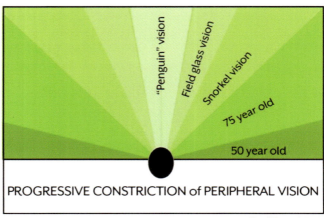

© Cloud Conrad, 2020.

2 | COGNITIVE FUNCTION and the SIGNALS of DECLINE

information available to him while wearing the cone. Do you wonder why he doesn't like it?

Some loss in peripheral vision is normal as we age. However as dementia progresses, a person's field of vision will become further restricted. In the early stages of dementia people get "snorkel vision" and, in the middle stages, binoculars or field glasses, and eventually, monocular vision[iv] like the single eyepiece worn by the "Penguin" of Batman® fame. This is a *substantial* reduction in field of vision, and it causes the person to be progressively less aware of the world around them via sight. Nine out of ten dementia patients will develop this monocular vision.[v]

By the time a person enters the middle stages of dementia, all that can be processed is within a space that is approximately 12 – 18 inches wide on all sides.[vi] Hold your arms out in front of you at about shoulder width and imagine only being able to see what was between your arms. You might easily startle a person with dementia if you approach them while outside their field of vision.

Another problem with this constriction is that depth perception is declining in the process. Depth perception is an important part of walking, navigating, and hand-eye coordination.

Loss of depth perception might make a person seem clumsier than usual. Knocking things over or tripping frequently may suggest the need for eyeglasses, or something more – a signal of decline in performance of visual processes of the occipital lobe.

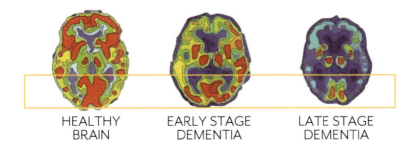

HEALTHY BRAIN   EARLY STAGE DEMENTIA   LATE STAGE DEMENTIA

Notice the amount of red, orange and yellow on the PET scans above – they shift from scan to scan, indicating a progressive cognitive decline.

2 | COGNITIVE FUNCTION and the SIGNALS of DECLINE

Compare the amount of red from scan to scan above. The loss of function, as illustrated here by decreasing brain activity, is creating any problems that seem vision-related.

VISUAL PROCESSING SUMMARY

Region	Occipital Lobe
Responsibility	Processes what the eyes take in
Specific Skills	Detecting form Detecting motion Detecting color Detecting depth Peripheral vision
Signals of Decline	Loss of peripheral vision Problems with object or facial recognition Problems distinguishing colors Light, shadow, reflection are confusing Loss of depth perception Motion blindness

NOTES

AUDITORY PROCESSING

Put your index fingers on your temples. The left and right temporal lobes are found inside your skull, beneath where your fingers are located. Both lobes are responsible for the processing of auditory data (what we hear) but the specific functions each contributes are different.

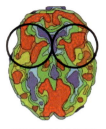

TEMPORAL LOBES

LINGUISTIC PROCESSING

We process linguistic data in the left temporal lobe. It is where vocabulary is stored, where we comprehend the meaning in others' speech and where speech production occurs – the assembly of words in a way that others can derive our intended message.

Having received a verbal message, all seniors tend to slow a little in response time to process and comprehend that, formulate a response, and then articulate that response. This is because working memory peaked years ago.

SIGNALS OF DECLINE

If showing signs of dementia in the left temporal lobe, a person will usually have a noticeably slower response time compared to his or her peers. It may seem like hearing loss to others.

As the left temporal lobe declines a person will typically have problems finding the right word. The "tip of the tongue" phenomenon is a normal hiccup in conversation for everyone. But with impairment a person loses the ability to retrieve the necessary word from their left temporal lobe. They will stop mid-sentence, unable to maintain their train of thought or unable to access, or form, the words of their response.

Nouns and pronouns seem to be more elusive than verbs and adjectives when word loss is a problem. Sometimes the lost word is someone's name, even though the unnamed person is recognized. Usually the person signaling this type of cognitive decline has the ability to find a verb to describe what the unnamed person is doing, on an adjective to describe how they look. This type of problem typically presents fairly early in the progression of dementia. If you observe this in a loved one, it may be a signal of decline.

When the left lobe is in decline, a person will also develop new problems completing sentences. Putting words together in a meaningful way, that effectively communicates a message to the listener, becomes challenging.

Reduced skill in comprehension of someone else's message will also take place. This will create misunderstandings that can escalate to arguments with family or harsh words to a sales person, for example.

When communication problems increase, they are accompanied by gradual social withdrawal. You will notice a decreased interest in routine outings to join friends. One-on-one exchanges become preferred because it is easier to avoid frustration or embarrassment when there is only one other person in the conversation.

As if this word loss is not challenging enough, other stimuli make linguistic processing even harder. Background noise in crowded places, lots of movement, many faces and other distractions can easily become overwhelming. The anxiety created by communication challenges, even in familiar places, can cause people with cognitive impairment to disengage from others. They may also disengage from hobbies that have a social aspect, like playing golf or participating in a book club, or holding seasonal tickets to sports or cultural events.

When dementia is present, the left temporal lobe will begin to decline first whereas the right temporal lobe will retain skills far longer. This is evident in the illustration on the following page.

Note the difference in color between the left and right temporal lobes in the three scans. There is progressively less activity in both left and right temporal lobes, however there is noticeably more activity on the right side, distinguished by the presence of comparatively warmer hues than the left.

2 | COGNITIVE FUNCTION and the SIGNALS of DECLINE

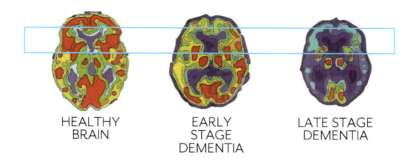

HEALTHY BRAIN   EARLY STAGE DEMENTIA   LATE STAGE DEMENTIA

LINGUISTIC PROCESSING SUMMARY

Region	Left Temporal Lobe
Responsibility	Linguistic communication
Specific Skills	Vocabulary Composing meaningful messages Comprehending meaning from others' messages
Signals of Decline	Slower response times Word loss, especially names of people and objects Inability to complete a sentence Starting the same sentence multiple times Trouble understanding others Social withdrawal

NOTES

3 RHYTHMIC and SONIC PROCESSING

Whereas the left temporal lobe is concerned with language, the right side is where rhythm skills– rhyming, music, poetry, prayer, rhythmic sound, and social chit chat[vii] – are performed.

What is social chit chat? It's the mindless conversations we have in which nothing of substance is said. Talk about the weather, how time flies, or how the holiday decorations seem to appear earlier and earlier in stores each year – these are great examples of social chit chat.

There's a rhythm to language and rhythm is central to speech. Social chit chat rides on the skirts of these rhythms.

"Hey, how are you?"

"I'm great, how are you? It's been so long!"

"It has been a long time – the kids keep us so busy!"

"You've got one off to college in the fall, right?"

"Yes, doesn't time fly?"

"Gone in a flash!"

"Well, good to see you!"

"Uh, huh. Good to see you too."

"Enjoy this weather!"

"Yes, aren't we blessed?"

It's really nothing talk. We do it our whole adult lives. We can practically carry on these conversations in our sleep.

Have you ever asked a question, received an answer, and then received an unexpected reaction when you followed through on that answer? Why was that? Perhaps the other person was leaning on social chit chat, especially intonation, volume and rate of

2 | COGNITIVE FUNCTION and the SIGNALS of DECLINE

speech, to comprehend the meaning of the conversation, rather than the words themselves.

A person with dementia will lose the formal language skills earlier, and more devastatingly, than rhythmic and sonic interpretive skills.[viii] A person retains skill on the right side for much longer in the progression of cognitive decline.

When the left temporal lobe starts to decline, the right temporal lobe will take over. One common scenario is that the person you are assisting has lost the ability to fully comprehend what you are asking them, but because he or she has retained the rhythm of language, you will get a "yes" or "no" answer.

It's an automatic response mechanism for people with dementia. They understand that you asked a question – they can see it in your face, hear it in your inflection. But they are just responding, neither really understanding nor answering, knowing from a lifetime of social interaction that questions deserve responses.

People with dementia show increasing reliance on social chit chat[ix] to get through conversations that are far more complex, making it seem as though they are following along. Because they are responding predictably to the mindless chatter of social chit chat, you believe they understand – that you are both on the same page. Therefore, frequent misunderstandings are a signal that the right temporal lobe is compensating for loss in the left temporal lobe.

Repeated use of "go to" phrases may support those with left temporal lobe decline as they convey their message. My step-father would say *"I'm just a poor country boy tryin' to get along."* This was his way of trying to shrug off the symptoms he displayed to others. It was his way of saying, *"I'm doing pretty well, given the situation. Please excuse me."*

DID HE REALLY SAY *THAT*?

There's one more important thing to know about the right temporal lobe. Forbidden words are stored here.

Most of us probably learned as young children that certain words were bad and not to be used in public, or not to be used at all!

27

Wash-your-mouth-out bad. In order to avoid a punishment, we didn't store these words with our "good" vocabulary.

But we didn't discard them either. We just moved them to the right side of our brain along with poetry, prayer and song. [x]

Use of lewd, mean or other inappropriate language is a signal that cognitive impairment is affecting language. When a person loses the good words, the bad ones seem like a fine replacement.

RHYTHMIC-SONIC PROCESSING SUMMARY

Region	Right Temporal Lobe
Responsibility	Rhythm and sound
Specific Skills	Poetry Prayer Song Social chit chat Bad words
Signals of Decline	Bad words and hate speech emerge with loss of vocabulary in left temporal lobe Social chit chat gives false sense of comprehension Reliance on "go to" phrases as filler words and dialogue responses

NOTES

2 | COGNITIVE FUNCTION and the SIGNALS of DECLINE

4 EXECUTIVE FUNCTION

The pre-frontal cortex is located in the front of our brain, behind the forehead. "Executive thinking" takes place here, specifically allowing us to see things from another person's point of view, compare and contrast things, weigh consequences, make decisions, and control our impulses. It's where we plan things and also where we start, sequence and stop actions. In humans this is the last part of the brain to develop.

It is normal to experience some decline in this area with age. From time to time we might miss a bill payment, or exhibit a lack of self-control. This is normal aging.

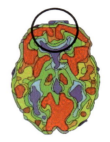

PRE-FRONTAL CORTEX

But when such lapses occur on a daily basis, cognitive decline may exist. Decline in this area creates an inability to sequence tasks, even familiar ones like writing a check or personal grooming. Did you know there are more than 30 steps to shaving your face? What about sorting, folding and putting away clean laundry? A lack of interest in personal grooming or housekeeping could be due to the challenge of executing multi-step processes.

Problems with sequencing may make it difficult to follow the well-worn process of preparing a known-by-heart recipe from scratch, like mother's skillet cornbread. "Broken" remotes, answering machines, printers, and cell phones may be signals of decline. Blaming the machine for malfunctioning may be an attempt to cover up the inability to execute multi-step processes.

Frontotemporal dementia, or FTD, involves pronounced impairment of the pre-frontal lobe. FTD has a notable correlation to early or young onset dementias.[xi] Because it starts affecting daily life much earlier than other dementias, signals of cognitive decline often start to reveal themselves in a person's forties or fifties.

Although it is tempting to attribute lack of self-control, strange behavior, and poor choice-making to a "mid-life" crisis, it may be

29

that something more serious is causing such sudden and nonsensical choices. Mid-life crisis is often the only other likely explanation to erratic or eccentric behavior.

A surprising, but true, example is the case of a prominent, 50-something physician who purchased a brand new helicopter (and flying lessons) on whim.[xii] When he continued to make other extraordinary "mid-life crises" type choices it became clear that frontotemporal dementia was to blame.

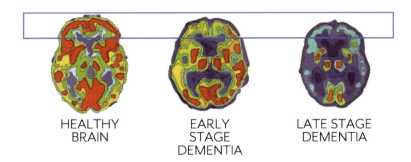

HEALTHY BRAIN   EARLY STAGE DEMENTIA   LATE STAGE DEMENTIA

Other executive-related signals of cognitive decline include the inability to experience empathy for others, inappropriate behavior, problems choosing among multiple options, **and the inability to delay gratification.**

EXECUTIVE FUNCTION SUMMARY

Region	Pre-frontal Lobe
Responsibility	Logic
Specific Skills	Comparison, analysis Weighing consequences, making decisions Planning and following plans Inhibition and self-control Empathy

2 | COGNITIVE FUNCTION and the SIGNALS of DECLINE

Signals of Decline	Taking much longer to complete regular tasks Difficulty making choices Poor decisions that seem like mid-life crisis Loss of "filters" that lead to inappropriate or over-disclosures Lack of inhibition/inappropriate behavior

NOTES
_____
_____
_____
_____
_____
_____
_____
_____
_____
_____
_____

SENSORY - MOTOR FUNCTION

Sensory processing and voluntary movement both occur in the parietal lobe. The parietal lobe is located between the occipital lobe and the frontal lobe, above the limbic system.

Imagine wearing a yarmulke or skullcap used for religious services. The parietal lobe is, roughly speaking, beneath the area covered by the skullcap.

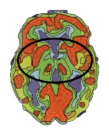

PARIETAL LOBE

Sensory and motor functions work in tandem. These brain skills seem to remain intact for a longer period of time for the person affected by dementia than other skills, however they are also affected.

2 | COGNITIVE FUNCTION and the SIGNALS of DECLINE

5 SENSORY FUNCTION

As for the sensory aspects, tactile sensation – identifying objects by touch, texture, weight, and contours – is registered in this part of the brain. So is taste.

Spatial relationships are understood here – that is, detecting existing relationships such as objects at rest as well as anticipating future relationships such as the trajectory of objects in motion.

This is where we get a sense of our body in space. The term for this awareness of our positioning relative to other objects and spaces around us is proprioception. [xiii]

Proprioception involves our muscles and tendons, primarily. Humans largely relate to our environment based on our major joints – shoulders, elbows, wrists, hips, knees, and ankles – which mark the perimeters of our bodies.

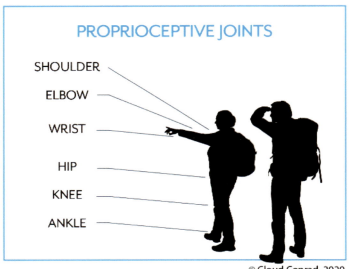

© Cloud Conrad, 2020.

Signals from these areas help us to separate our bodies from the adjacent negative space or objects. Clumsiness will result when the sense of the body in space is impaired by dementia.

32

2 | COGNITIVE FUNCTION and the SIGNALS of DECLINE

This part of the brain is also responsible for the detection of pain. The inability to detect and/or locate pain will occur as dementia progresses. This may cause a person to act in a way that is atypical for their personality, which can be a signal that the person is actually experiencing physical pain, yet is unable to detect and/or convey it to others.

The perception of pain may have been masked or generalized and the person couldn't connect the pain to a cause. There are often unexpected outbursts caused by this hindrance.

Dementia's progression also causes limitations in taste sensation. The ability to detect and distinguish taste will decrease, especially the umami, or savory, taste response. [xiv] For people with dementia other taste sensations seem to remain longer than others. Sweets are one example. My father became a loyal devotee of Moose Tracks® ice cream. Alcohol, another sugar, is something to which people with dementia may be drawn.

Smell is not processed in this area (it's processed by the olfactory gland and covered in upcoming pages).

SENSORY PROCESSING SUMMARY

Region	Parietal Lobe
Responsibility	Interpret sensations from the body
Specific Skills	Receiving sensory stimuli and calling for a response Position of body in space via proprioceptors
Signals of Decline	Inability to detect pain Clumsiness Food preferences become limited in range

NOTES

2 | COGNITIVE FUNCTION and the SIGNALS of DECLINE

6 MOTOR FUNCTION

Voluntary movement – what we consciously tell our bodies to do – requires the use of spatial and proprioception data to support physical movement, or motor function. The parietal lobe governs hand-eye coordination and fine motor skills. It also uses information from our emotion centers, covered later, to make facial expressions.

As dementia progresses, muscle memory will tend to remain intact for a long while. Yet manual dexterity – the ability to execute the motor sequence – will deteriorate sooner.

Loss of gross and fine motor skills are results of decline in this functional area. You may notice general clumsiness or trouble with hand-eye coordination.

It is normal for handwriting to change with age. However with dementia handwriting will become increasingly difficult to interpret and gradually deteriorate to illegible scratching if this deterioration signals dementia. Illegible handwriting will be compounded by the inability to compose coherent phrases and sentences and put them down on paper. Fastening buttons, snaps and zippers, and tying shoelaces will become more difficult as impairment advances.

Slowed movement is also a signal of cognitive decline related to sensory/motor processing. Related issues involve mumbling or slurred speech and shuffling.

VOLUNTARY MOTION SUMMARY

Region	Parietal Lobe
Responsibility	Intentional movement

2 | COGNITIVE FUNCTION and the SIGNALS of DECLINE

Specific Skills	Responding to sensory stimuli with motion Hand-eye coordination Gross motor skills Fine motor skills
Signals of Decline	Mumbling/poor enunciation Illegible handwriting Trouble with fasteners like buttons, snaps, zippers, and shoelaces Shuffling when walking

NOTES

SELF-PRESERVATION

The hippocampus is closer to the center of our skulls in a complex part of the brain called the limbic system, in the medial temporal lobe. The limbic system is responsible for self-preservation.

The hippocampus contributes to self-preservation by providing humans capability for intentional adaptation. A chief way this happens is through associative thinking, specifically new learning and memory formation. The other way is through our survival instincts.

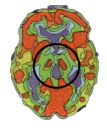

MEDIAL TEMPORAL LOBE

2 | COGNITIVE FUNCTION and the SIGNALS of DECLINE

7 NEW LEARNING & MEMORY

The hippocampus is where we form new memories. It's where we learn new information. It's part of the limbic system, responsible for human survival.

The caveman survived by learning and retaining new information long enough to use it. A caveman might have noticed that the wildebeests seemed to congregate by a particular shoal on the river bank at the same time each afternoon. That might be useful to know when trying to feed his family.

Sense of time and place is understood in the hippocampus. This helped the caveman notice the pattern of behavior demonstrated by the wildebeests, gathering at these shoals when the sun was just so in the sky.

The hippocampus is also responsible for wayfinding, so our caveman could find this special location on the next afternoon when he returned with his spear. Inability to navigate familiar paths or routes, such as to the grocery store or mall, is a signal that dementia is present. The brain does not connect the different scenery or imagery encountered along the path to the old memories of where to turn and when to proceed forward. Each scene or city block, perhaps, is effectively a new learning.

Dementia creates loss of immediate recall, including recent events and new information. Although seniors normally misplace items – we all do – a signal of cognitive decline would be having a hard time keeping track of objects such as phone, keys, and wallet. Loss of immediate recall will also challenge a person to be able to keep up with a conversation.

Another sign that the hippocampus is declining include missed appointments, and misplaced objects caused by the inability to retain new learning and/or trouble keeping track of time.

Seniors do become a little forgetful – that's normal. But a major signal that new information is not retained – that a new memory was not formed – is repetitive questions.

36

2 | COGNITIVE FUNCTION and the SIGNALS of DECLINE

The hippocampus is one of the early areas to be affected by dementia. In fact "forgetfulness" is usually the first signal that there may be a cognitive health issue.

When newer memories become subordinate to older memories, a person with dementia may be confused by the present "you" because it does not match up with *their* sense of your identify – an identity defined by the past. Since you no longer wear your hair in braids as you did in the 1970's, you cannot possibly be the same woman your husband married years ago. You may become unrecognizable without these markers from the past. Or, your identity may seem to come and go for the person with dementia.

Although episodic memories get lost (the facts surrounding past events), emotional memories (the feelings surrounding those events) remain.[xv] This is why caregivers should focus on emotions, not facts, particularly in times when symptoms escalate.

NEW LEARNING & MEMORY SUMMARY

Region	Hippocampus (part of the limbic system), in the Medial Temporal Lobe
Responsibility	Survival by intentional adaptation
Specific Skills	Formation of new memories, new learning Immediate recall Control over stored memories Sense of time and place
Signals of Decline	Repetitive questions Inability to follow directions, way-finding Difficulty remembering new information Misplacing things, inability to retrace steps Missed appointments

NOTES

2 | COGNITIVE FUNCTION and the SIGNALS of DECLINE

8 SURVIVAL INSTINCTS

The amygdalae are also part of the limbic system. Positioned next to the hippocampus, the amygdalae drive our survival instincts. When we detect danger, it is the amygdalae that drives our "fight or flight" response. In this way, with the hippocampus, the amygdalae drives emotions.

While watching the wildebeests congregate by the river shoal, our caveman heard the rustling in the bushes behind him, He knew it was a saber tooth tiger but he turned around anyway, needing to see it to be sure. He knew he was in danger.

Should he spear the saber tooth or run like bloody hell? The amygdalae would decide. While he experienced that sense of danger, the caveman's adrenaline surged, a biological response that would protect him, powering his motion, however he chose to respond – whether by stab or by stride.

Being less and less able to interpret the world around them and therefore more often surprised by it and less able to respond to it, a person living with dementia faces a constant sense of threat. Chronic elevated anxiety is the result. The frustration of not being able to do as before, to cope as before, also triggers escalated symptoms of dementia.

In the illustration that follows, notice that the two round red areas highlighted seem to get bigger and more pronounced, whereas in every other function's progressive detail, the red areas seem to diminish over time. What this suggests is that the person with dementia has a fight-or-flight mechanism that is constantly on alert.

38

2 | COGNITIVE FUNCTION and the SIGNALS of DECLINE

This will cause them to have feelings of vulnerability – to feel easily threatened.

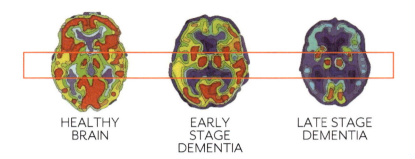

HEALTHY BRAIN   EARLY STAGE DEMENTIA   LATE STAGE DEMENTIA

This is understandable, considering a person with dementia has fewer pieces of information available to them that would ordinarily be processed by all of the other brain functions we've discussed – information that might help them survive. They also have fewer tools to communicate these threats or the associated emotions.

Most escalations are due in part to the amygdalae functioning in overdrive. In this high anxiety state, facts aren't facts. There is no reasoning with a person with dementia in this state. Logic does not apply. The person is solely interested in defending himself or herself from the unreal, but *perceived*, threat. Delusions are a signal of dementia.

As we get older, we become attached to our routines. We enjoy the familiar. When things don't go as planned, we might become edgy, even grumpy. However, we can recover, devise a "Plan B" and move on with the alternative.

Thrown off, and in a state of high anxiety, a person signaling symptoms of dementia will have an inability to "move on" when things don't go as expected. They cannot devise a Plan B themselves nor can they entertain your Plan B. It is hard to re-direct them to a calmer topic.

The amygdalae is where our pleasure center is located, as well as our safety awareness. Protective sensations like "I'm cold" or "I'm

2 | COGNITIVE FUNCTION and the SIGNALS of DECLINE

thirsty" as well as permissive gratifications like "I want candy" are functions of the amygdalae.

Previously you learned that odor isn't part of sensory processing in the parietal lobe. In fact the olfactory gland is located next to the amygdalae. In prehistoric days, the scent of a saber tooth tiger upwind would be an important cue for survival of the caveman.

Given the close proximity of olfactory processing and survival instincts in the brain, it seems no coincidence that smells conjure associative emotions. We all experience certain smells that bring a wave of emotions – a certain perfume, or the smell of your grandmother's house. The smell of Thanksgiving dinner cooking *should* summon pleasant emotions like fellowship and satiation. Hopefully such aromas are *not* a cue that your survival is threatened!

Some studies suggest that people living with dementia cannot smell peanut butter or that loss of various smells is a very early sign.[xvi] This may not be universally true, and this theory is under-researched, but it proved true in my father's case.

SURVIVAL INSTINCTS SUMMARY

Region	Amygdalae (part of the limbic system), in the Medial Temporal Lobe
Responsibility	Survival by defense
Specific Skills	Detecting and responding to threat With the hippocampus, forming emotions Pleasure seeking
Signals of Decline	Heightened sense of urgency Inability to delay gratification Distrust, paranoia, delusions Over-reaction when things go wrong Becoming upset makes other brain function worse Aggression, agitation, combativeness, anxiety

2 | COGNITIVE FUNCTION and the SIGNALS of DECLINE

NOTES

CONCLUSION

The differences between normal aging and changes that might be cause for concern have been laid out based on eight key brain functions. We have also discussed how changes in the brain, attributed to aging which is not normal, will display as signals of cognitive decline.

You may have been dismayed to notice one or more of these signals, either in yourself or someone close to you. Is it really a sign of cognitive decline to display these signals? There are three gauges to apply to this question in order to know for sure.

IS IT NOT AS IT USED TO BE?

If it is different for that person, and not like before, it may be cause for concern.[xvii] If the person of concern has always had trouble presenting themselves well, with a low bar for personal grooming and dressing, then he wouldn't notice or mind a permanent stain on his lapel. If however, the person has always been fabulously coiffed and fastidiously dressed but now doesn't seem to pay much attention to appearance, it is likely a signal of cognitive decline.

2 | COGNITIVE FUNCTION and the SIGNALS of DECLINE

IS IT JUST A "SENIOR MOMENT" OR IS IT SOMETHING MORE?

When there is a lost word or a forgotten appointment, do they eventually reclaim the word or the person's name? Or manage to remember the dentist appointment in time to show up? If the answer is no, this may be more than normal aging.

DOES IT INTERRUPT THE FLOW OF DAILY LIVING?

Is the problem infrequent, or frequent enough that it happens daily and causes more than mere inconvenience or embarrassment? If these moments have become part of daily living, it is likely cause for concern.[xviii]

FIELD ASSIGNMENT:

ASSESSMENT EXERCISE: Complete the Signals of Cognitive Decline Assessment found in Appendix B.

Use the knowledge gained in Chapter Two about aging, cognitive decline and signals of possible impairment to complete this assignment. The **Signals of Cognitive Decline Assessment** probes 30 potential changes in cognitive functions that may signal a cause for concern. Use the **Wheel of Cognitive Function & Decline** found in Appendix A as a supporting visual while comparing each of the cognitive functions to your observations.

It is an introspective exercise to help create clarity on the observations you've made about the memory, thinking, and actions of someone close to you. *This assessment is not to be construed as a medical diagnostic tool.*

As you work through the assessment, keep in mind that one need not show all 30 potential signals in order for there to be reason to seek medical advice. Even one signal is cause for concern.[xix] That said, many of these signals may also be symptoms of depression or other, treatable disorders and do not necessarily point to dementia.

2 | COGNITIVE FUNCTION and the SIGNALS of DECLINE

[i] Hartshorne, J. K., & Germine, L.T. (2015, April). When does cognitive functioning peak? The asynchronous rise and fall of different cognitive abilities across the life span. *Psychological Science, 26*(4), 433-443.

[ii] This illustration and the others in our series were created by Camille Hayes to represent a set of PET scans published online and credited to Gary W. Small, MD, of the UCLA School of Medicine. The artwork was commissioned by the author in order to create an original, clear representation of the scans. The locations of individual brain lobes and functions are approximate.

[iii] MedBridge (2016, July 25). *Dementia video: Changes in vision – Teepa Snow | MedBridge* [Video]. YouTube. https://www.youtube.com/watch?v=iaUsRa5kNyw

[iv] Snow, T. (2012). *Dementia Caregiver Guide*. Cedar Village Retirement Community.

[v] Snow (2012)

[vi] Home Care Assistance. (2020). How vision changes with dementia. *HomeCareAssistance*. https://homecareassistance.com/e-books/dementia-care-guide/how-vision-changes-with-dementia

[vii] Teepa Snow's Positive Approach to Care (2017, December 21) *How dementia affects language skills*. [Video]. YouTube. https://www.youtube.com/watch?v=0BlZF_4EKp4

[viii] Teepa Snow's Positive Approach to Care (2017)

[ix] Teepa Snow's Positive Approach to Care (2017)

[x] Teepa Snow's Positive Approach to Care (2017)

[xi] Lee, S. MD. (2020). Frontotemporal dementia: Clinical features and diagnosis. *UpToDate*. Retrieved September 22, 2020, from https://www.uptodate.com/contents/frontotemporal-dementia-clinical-features-and-diagnosis

[xii] Castaneda, R. (2019, April 18). What is frontotemporal dementia? *US News & World Report*. https://health.usnews.com/health-care/patient-advice/articles/what-is-frontotemporal-dementia

[xiii] Williams, L. (2018, June 18). Proprioception: Making sense of body position. *VeritasHealth*. https://www.sports-health.com/sports-injuries/general-injuries/proprioception-making-sense-body-position

[xiv] Kouzuki, M., Ichikawa, J., Shirasagi, D. et al. (2020, March 26). Detection and recognition thresholds for five basic tastes in patients with mild cognitive impairment and Alzheimer's disease dementia. *BMC Neurol* 20, 110. https://doi.org/10.1186/s12883-020-01691-7

[xv] Harvard Health Letter. (2007, January). The emotional side of Alzheimer's disease. *HealthHarvard*. https://www.health.harvard.edu/newsletter_article/the-emotional-side-of-alzheimers-disease

[xvi] Wood, J. (2018, August 5). Loss of smell can predict cognitive decline in the elderly. *PsychCentral*. https://psychcentral.com/news/2017/09/30/loss-of-smell-can-predict-cognitive-decline-in-elderly/126715.html

2 | COGNITIVE FUNCTION and the SIGNALS of DECLINE

[xvii] Alzheimer's Association. (2020) 10 Warning Signs. *Alzheimer's Association*. [Video]. https://training.alz.org/products/4062/10-warning-signs-of-alzheimers?_ga=2.39326627.1894699948.1600821175-573432083.1578076153

[xviii] Alzheimer's Association (2020)

[xix] Alzheimer's Association (2020)

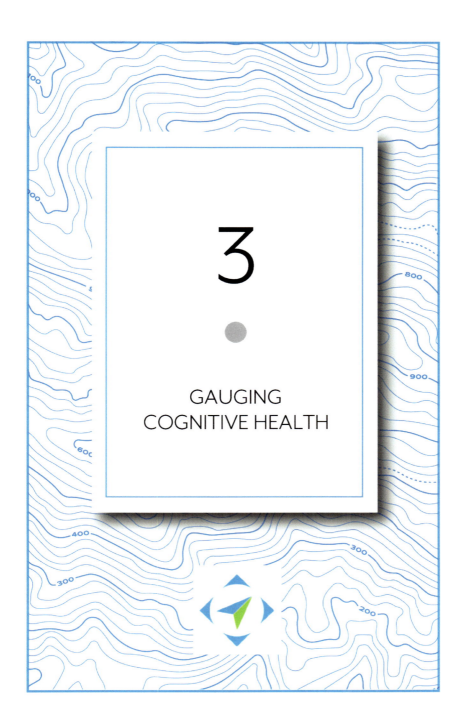

3

GAUGING COGNITIVE HEALTH

3 | GAUGING COGNITIVE HEALTH

> For years, Karen has spent lunchtime on Wednesdays in a lively but friendly Canasta rivalry with three other women. Karen had been the one to "discover" Canasta in high school. She taught Bea, Louise and Cindy how to play and score. A longstanding friendship developed over the cards. And lately, Karen can't keep track of the score. Bea, Karen's partner, has noticed Karen's problems adding up her points correctly. She asks several times per hand, *"What's the score again?"* Exasperated, Bea cried out last week, *"Why can't you keep up? What's your problem??"* It didn't go well. Yesterday, Karen called Cindy to suggest they find a substitute for today's game, feigning a stomach bug. In truth, she was aware of her problems with scoring and embarrassed they showed outwardly.

Depression can make it difficult to complete tasks or focus for any length of time. Thyroid problems can create confusion and forgetfulness, also affecting a person's ability to focus, to learn new information and to recall it promptly.

Lyme disease can cause significant short term memory loss. Prescription drugs, hot flashes, fatty diets, vitamin deficiencies, and a higher "infectious burden" can also cause memory problems.[i] Karen's condition will eventually be diagnosed as

> *It's easy to confuse certain chronic conditions with dementia.*

hypothyroidism and she will be treated. But unfortunately, *she missed more Wednesdays than necessary worrying that she had dementia before seeking any medical opinion.*

ASSESSING COGNITIVE DECLINE

It's easy to confuse certain chronic conditions with dementia. Physical, mental, and cognitive and health are interwoven, yet interdependent. This is a major reason why early attention is so important. Any opportunity to identify a condition that is potentially reversible should be taken.

MAPPING THE TERRAIN

Using the Field Assignment at the end of Chapter Two – the **Signals of Cognitive Decline Assessment** in Appendix B – we will bring your key findings into focus so that you may survey the land

3 | GAUGING COGNITIVE HEALTH

around you and determine your present position. *Table 3.1: Cognitive Health Gauge* will support you as you review your Assessment findings and formulate your conclusions.

PLOTTING YOUR LOCATION

As we explore the possibility of decline in someone we know, a snapshot of this moment in time is helpful. Below, we'll gauge the composite cognitive landscape to capture his or her baseline.

Beneath each of the cognitive functions in **Table 3.1: Cognitive Health Gauge**, write the sub-total of points scored for that function on the Signals Assessment. On the right, place a circle inside the box with the point value that is closest to your subtotal. Round up or down as necessary. (Example: If the subtotal for the Sample section is 23, place the circle in the box above 25 as follows.)

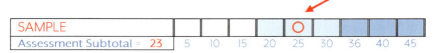

After completing the table add the date in the space provided.

TABLE 3.1: COGNITIVE HEALTH GAUGE

	NO ACTION	MONITOR	CONCERN
VISUAL Assessment Subtotal =	5 10 15	20 25 30	36 40 45
LINGUISTIC Assessment Subtotal =	8 16 24	32 40 48	56 64 72
EXECUTIVE Assessment Subtotal =	4 8 12	16 20 24	28 32 36
SENSORY-MOTOR Assessment Subtotal =	5 10 15	20 25 30	36 40 45
LEARNING/NEW MEMORY Assessment Subtotal =	4 8 12	16 20 24	28 32 36
SURVIVAL Assessment Subtotal =	4 8 12	16 20 24	28 32 36

Date of Assessment

3 | GAUGING COGNITIVE HEALTH

The unshaded boxes (the three on the left of each row, indicate no cause for concern. The lightly shaded areas suggest that close monitoring is the minimum response. And the darkly shaded areas point to the need for medical advice.

Where are your circles relative to each other and to the shaded regions? What insights does this visual display trigger?

IF IT'S NORMAL AGING

"This doesn't apply to me right now," you may be thinking. Your findings using the Signals of Cognitive Decline Assessment in Appendix B may have brought you to the conclusion that you are observing normal aging processes in your loved one.

There may be no cause for concern and no action necessary. If this is your view at present, what you've learned about the cognitive functions and their decline is something you can continue to use to remain alert and aware of brain health over time.

Because aging is the primary risk factor for dementia, the passing of time necessitates monitoring cognitive health at regular intervals just as with cardiac, reproductive, and dental health. Completing the Assessment, you will be well-equipped to be attentive for these signals in your family members, and even yourself, as time advances.

Going forward, use this gauge periodically to take quick "check-ins" of the present moment in time and compare each to prior times. These quick checks should be completed two or three times a year.

When making theses updates, add a new circle to Table 3.1 on any rows where you have noticed a functional change since the last time you checked. *(HINT: By using different ink colors as you do these quick checks you can easily capture and detect the progression of your findings over time on this one table.)*

The **Cognitive Health Gauge** (Table 3.1) displays a bird's eye view of the contours of the individual's cognitive landscape as well as any changes as time advances. As we explore the subject of decline

3 | GAUGING COGNITIVE HEALTH

in a loved one, it will be useful to have this visual depiction and know the dates associated with any changes in the topography.

Record the date of each scheduled update in the spaces provided in **Table 3.2: Tracking Cognitive Health Schedule**, to maintain regular "check in" intervals. Add these dates to your calendar.

TABLE 3.2: TRACKING COGNITIVE HEALTH SCHEDULE

TRACKING COGNITIVE HEALTH SCHEDULE	
Update on	*Update on*
Update on	*Update on*
Update on	*Update on*

IF IT'S CAUSE FOR CONCERN

In the scenario where signals create cause for concern, what you know about your loved one will shape your response to your conclusions. You may already have a sense of whether he or she is aware of the changes to their thinking, feelings, and actions beyond what appears to be just senior moments.

His or her awareness doesn't necessarily make your dialog about cognitive health easier. Denial, compensation, and covering are likely companions on this stretch of road if signs of dementia exist.

WHAT HAVE YOU NOTICED?

The Signals of Cognitive Decline Assessment, Appendix B, aided you in identifying any areas where concern is warranted. It will be helpful to bring those signals from Appendix B into this section so that it's all on one page for a succinct reference point. To do this, use The Signals of Cognitive Decline Inventory found in Table 3.3 on the following page.

3 | GAUGING COGNITIVE HEALTH

TABLE 3.3: SIGNALS OF COGNITIVE DECLINE INVENTORY

Place a check in the box to the right of each signal below that scored five or higher on the Signals of Cognitive Decline Assessment.

VISUAL	Problems with object or facial recognition	
	Objects hide in plain sight	
	Startled by shadow, reflection, or other eye trickery	
	Challenges with depth perception	
	Seeing things that aren't actually there/hallucinations	
LINGUISTIC	Word loss	
	Apparent loss of thought mid-sentence	
	Slower response times when answering	
	Social withdrawal	
	Repetitive phrases	
	Misunderstandings	
	Unexpected outbursts	
	Inappropriate language	
EXECUTIVE	Inappropriate behavior	
	Problems planning	
	Inability to make decisions/problems choosing	
	Trouble with familiar tasks	
SENSORY OR MOTOR	Slowed movement	
	Inability to detect pain	
	Mumbling/poor enunciation	
	Illegible handwriting	
	Problems with fasteners like zippers, buttons, shoelaces	
MEMORY, LEARNING	Getting lost on familiar paths or routes	
	Missed appointments	
	Repetitive questions	
	Misplaced items	
SURVIVAL	Delusions/believing things that aren't true	
	Inability to "move on" with Plan B	
	Heightened sense of urgency	
	Chronic, elevated anxiety	

3 | GAUGING COGNITIVE HEALTH

CHARTING YOU COURSE

You have now created two useful summaries of your observations as discovered in the Signals Assessment. *Table 3.1: Gauging Cognitive Health* provides an overview and timeline of cognitive functions potentially affected, and *Table 3.3: Signals of Cognitive Decline Inventory* highlights specific signals for each that deserve our attention. Between these two tools *you now have direct language to support you as you communicate any concerns.*

Chapter Four will help you develop an effective, empathetic approach to share your observations with the person for whom you have concerns. You'll actually script your lines and rehearse them with a partner. But before moving forward toward that objective, take a moment to do this field assignment to help you gain your bearings.

FIELD ASSIGNMENT:

JOURNAL EXERCISE: Bringing your concerns into focus.

From the Signals of Cognitive Decline Inventory, select the three signals that give you the greatest concern. Write those signals in the space provided at the top of each of the sections that follow. Then, answer the prompts for each of those signals.

Signal #1: _____
In what ways does this signal seem unusual, not as it used to be?
_____
_____
_____
_____

In what ways is it more than just a "senior moment"?
_____
_____
_____

3 | GAUGING COGNITIVE HEALTH

In what ways does it interrupt the flow of daily living?

Signal #2:

In what ways does this signal seem unusual, not as it used to be?

In what ways is it more than just a "senior moment"?

In what ways does it interrupt the flow of daily living?

Signal #3:

In what ways does this signal seem unusual, not as it used to be?

In what ways is it more than just a "senior moment"?

3 | GAUGING COGNITIVE HEALTH

In what ways does it interrupt the flow of daily living?

JOURNAL EXERCISE: Sharing your observations with family members.

Use this space to make notes about other key insights and observations not captured elsewhere. Include insights and observations from other family members with whom you may have discussed this topic.

3 | GAUGING COGNITIVE HEALTH

3 | GAUGING COGNITIVE HEALTH

[i] Melone, L. (2019). 8 unexpected things that mess with your memory. [Time Special Edition]. *The Science of Memory*. Meredith Publishing.

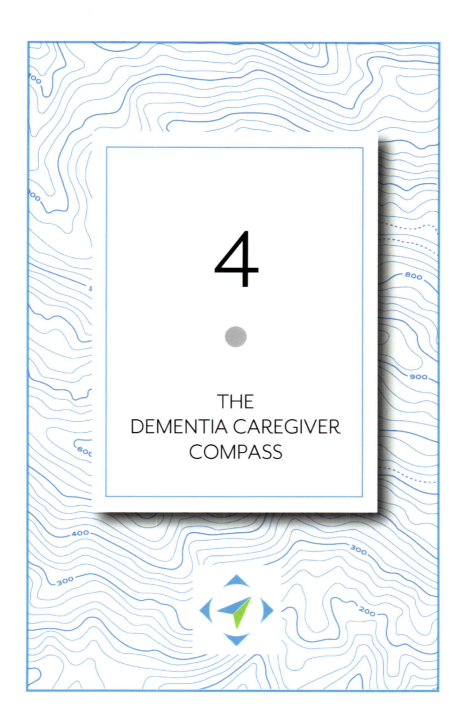

4

THE DEMENTIA CAREGIVER COMPASS

> Percy keeps the article, so carefully cut from the newspaper and neatly folded, in his wallet. *"Red Wine May Aid Memory, Study Found"* frequently sees daylight. He will pull it out and show it to Estelle when there is a silence at the table that needs filling. *"The doctor says that red wine is good for me,"* he will say, rolling over on one hip to reach for his wallet. Married forty-nine years, Percy and Estelle have a lot of wordless periods. He will produce the article several times in the course of a meal to repair the silence.

Unlike caregiving for a person battling cancer, you'll need a different set of bearings to travel the dementia caregiver's path. No other disease affects a person's thoughts, feelings, and actions like dementia. *You will not be able to interact with the person in your care in the same ways you would a person battling another form of degenerative disease or cancer.* In terrain you cannot yet chart, you will not reach your desired state without a proper orientation.

YOUR ORIENTATION IN CAREGIVING

The foundational principles of **The Dementia Caregiver Compass** are intended to help you find your bearings and set your direction in caregiving, in general *and* each time you approach the person in your care. On a physical journey you might consult your compass several times as you traverse steep inclines, thread narrow valleys, and circumvent natural or other barriers in your path. The compass helps you find your way, even at those points when your destination is not within your line of sight. Were you at sea, the compass would help you stay on course in the absence of landmarks to gauge your position and progress.

The compass is the most important tool in your travel pack

Without a compass you would lose your way, perhaps encounter badlands or predators. Such events would force you to respond to unnecessary adversity with a depleted supply of energy and provisions, perhaps never regaining course and arriving at your destination. A compass helps you stay on course to go the distance.

As a dementia caregiver, it's important to adjust your "settings". The Dementia Caregiver Compass can help you do that.

Dignity and trust

I see and hear of situations in which caregivers, with the best of intentions in mind, will do or say things that unnecessarily jeopardize the dignity of the person in their care and, in the process, the trust of the relationship between caregiver and person living with dementia. *If caregivers do not have the trust of the person in their care, then caregiving will always be uphill, where the air thins as altitude increases.* In caregiving, you need the person in your care to want to work with you. In order to do so, they will need to feel secure in your care. The key to that security is trust.

Other reference materials make the unfortunate mistake of likening people living with dementia to children. This is often used in the context of mental and physical ability but is especially common in difficult situations and often equated to the "acting out" of a child.

Viewing those living with dementia as child-like and exhibiting child-like behavior robs a person of their dignity. It is unhealthy for caregivers to perceive their loved one as a child-like being. Such a perception may erode trust and induce stressors that thwart forward progress toward the desired state of well-being and joy. The Dementia Caregiver Compass is a more effective orientation.

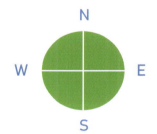

N – E – W – S: in CAREGIVING

Think of the four foundational principles of **The Dementia Caregiver Compass** as points on a compass. The North, East, West and South points on a true compass create a helpful acronym to remember the points on our Dementia Caregiver Compass.

As with all navigation, regardless of your direction of travel, the other points on the compass are just as important in setting your bearings as the point guiding you. In order to hike in a northeasterly direction, awareness of your relative position to all other directions is necessary. So, all points on The Dementia Caregiver Compass are of equal and simultaneous importance.

N STANDS FOR **NEEDS**

Humans are bonded by universal, essential needs. These needs do not diminish with age, or with dementia. These essentials span the gamut, from basic, tangible needs – food and shelter – to identity-based needs, like having a sense of belonging, self-worth, and purpose. These are essential needs for humans to survive and thrive.

In 1943, behavioral scientist Abraham Maslow published a theory we now know as Maslow's Hierarchy of Need. His research identified five universal, interdependent needs and ordered them by their relative importance. Maslow believed one would first need to have food, shelter and warmth before being able to pursue other, higher order needs.[i]

Other behavioral scientists have developed alternate theories that include additional needs and/or a balanced rather than hierarchical view of their importance. In spite of the variations to his theory, other scientists seem to recognize the five needs Maslow identified.

TABLE 4.1: MASLOW'S HIERARCHY OF NEED

Source: Abraham Maslow, PhD.

Sharing these universal human needs, a caregiver and their person are cast as equals. The needs to feel a sense of love and belonging, to contribute, and to have a sense of purpose are as strong for the person in your care as they are for you.

Unlike physiological and safety needs, the higher order needs refer to intangible aspects of our existence which shape our individual identity. These identity-based needs are as strong in late stage dementia as they were in the person's cognitive peak. This point is important in caregiving philosophically and, as you'll find out later in this Guide, practically as well.

E STANDS FOR EMOTIONS

Our identity-based needs are characterized and described on *emotional* terms. When we discuss specific cognitive functions later you'll learn that, as a person's dementia progresses, *facts eventually don't matter. But emotions always will.* That's because our senses of belonging, personal worth, and purpose are gauged by intangible, emotional measures rather than the finite, rational measures we use to gauge physiological and safety needs.

Most of the difficult situations that arise for caregivers are caused by an unmet human need. Needs may be physical, environmental, or emotional. All needs have emotions associated with them.

TABLE 4.2: EMOTIONS OF NEED

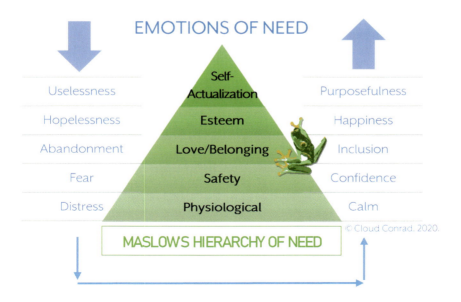

4 | THE DEMENTIA CAREGIVER COMPASS

The intention in caregiving is to transform the negative emotions associated with unmet needs into positive emotions. You will develop skills to address those unmet needs, using the knowledge and skills gained through The Guide.

W STANDS FOR WILL

Along with his or her needs, a person living with dementia retains a sense of will until the end stages of the disease. Will is the drive to meet our human needs. One can't simply *will* a thing to happen though. Without power and ability, nothing can be accomplished.

Dementia will destroy a person's power and ability to accomplish higher order tasks gradually, eventually impeding tasks of daily living. The imbalance of will, power, and ability is a constant source of stress for people with dementia because need fulfillment is uncertain at best.

S STANDS FOR SYMPTOMS

You'll likely come across reference material in your research that speaks of "challenging behaviors" caregivers face in their role. This is another example of troublesome terminology. *To think of the elevated situations that become trials for caregivers as "challenging behaviors" has some dangerous implications.*

> Symptoms of dementia are the root cause of challenging situations, not the person or the behavior.

When we think of these escalations as behaviors it invites a construct that involves correction or consequence. And, behaviors are by definition *chosen responses* to the stimuli around us, driven in large part by the personality of the person exhibiting the behavior.

Who is really challenged?
When dementia is present, at least two parts of that person's brain are dying.[ii] People living with dementia are using what is still available to them to communicate with us. *Incomplete information, slower processing, and a heightened sense of threat all serve to limit their choice in response or reaction.*

The signals that we first identify as signs of decline become symptoms as dementia advances in the brain. At times when needs are unmet, *dementia's symptoms may cause escalated situations.* Less and less often we see logical, conscious responses to our loved one's perceptions/interpretations of his or her world.

It would be dishonest to assert that escalated situations aren't challenging. But when we think of them as symptoms rather than challenging behaviors, it is easier to focus on and respond to the disease, which is the root cause of the problem, not the person or the behavior. *Escalated situations are driven by symptom-related behaviors rather than personality-related behaviors.*

For this reason, this Guide intentionally avoids the term "challenging behavior" and opts instead for an orientation that centers on the idea that dementia's *symptoms* are the source of escalations.

CONCLUSION

Armed with the Dementia Caregiver Compass, you are ready to set your direction and begin navigating your caregiver role. This role begins the moment you determine signals of cognitive decline exist. Whether or not these signals advance to Alzheimer's or other dementia, the orientation should be the same.

FIELD ASSIGNMENT:

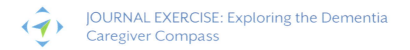

JOURNAL EXERCISE: Exploring the Dementia Caregiver Compass

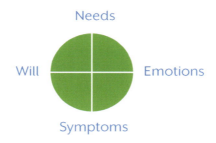

4 | THE DEMENTIA CAREGIVER COMPASS

Using the space that follows, record responses to the corresponding prompts.

Which points on the Dementia Caregiver Compass resonate most for you?

Think of a time when someone you know was unable to express an unmet need successfully, *whether related to cognitive issues or not.* How were they communicating their need to you?

What emotions seemed most prominent based on the interaction?

Did you recognize the unmet need? How did you respond?

_____
_____
_____
_____
_____

What worked AND/OR what would you have done differently in an attempt to transform negative emotion(s), if they existed, to positive ones?

_____
_____
_____
_____
_____
_____
_____
_____

Thinking about the person you are concerned for, consider each point on the Dementia Caregiver Compass and what you can bring from each principle as you anticipate having a conversation about cognitive health. Make some notes in the spaces provided below.

N – E – W – S

NEEDS

What is relevant from Maslow's theory of universal human needs as you prepare to address your concerns? How might you check your understanding of the unmet need(s) you identified? In what ways might you address these needs going forward?

_____
_____
_____
_____
_____
_____
_____
_____
_____
_____

EMOTIONS

There is a lot of opportunity for negative emotions to surface in such a delicate conversation. How will your awareness about human needs and emotions apply to your approach?

WILL

In what ways might the imbalance of will to power and ability introduce stressors in your conversation? What opportunities might exist to provide some choice to, or play to the remaining strengths of, the person for whom you are concerned?

SYMPTOMS

The signals you've noticed are potential symptoms. But unlike behaviors, symptoms don't invite corrections or consequences. In what ways does a supportive orientation differ from a corrective/combative one?

---

[i] Maslow, A. H. (1943). A theory of human motivation. *Psychological Review*, 50(4), 370-396.

[ii] Leonard, W. (2018, November 1). *What do you want to know about dementia?* .Healthline. https://www.healthline.com/health/dementia

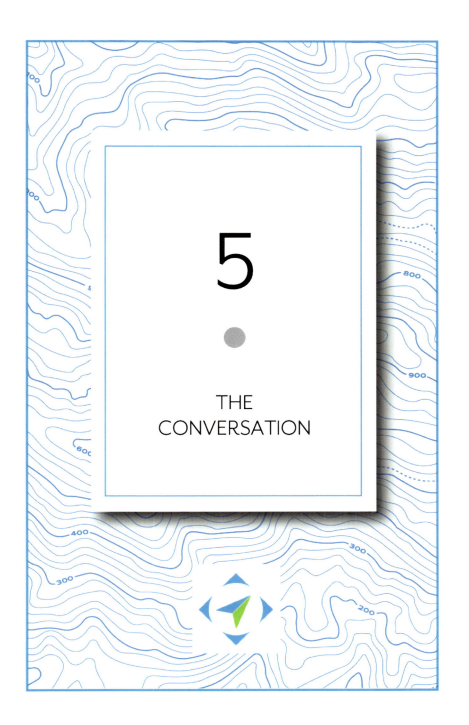

5

THE CONVERSATION

5 | THE CONVERSATION

> Marissa knows her mother is struggling in the kitchen. Last week, Marissa came through the back door to a pot of water, unattended, on the kitchen stove, boiled nearly dry. This was the second time this month. *"Mom??"* she yelled to an empty first floor. Her mother eventually rounded the corner, chatting away on the phone with busy, red lips that gave vivid contrast to the dried clay mask ghosting her face. But there was also the Father's Day incident. Mom made her grandmother's "secret recipe" gingerbread dessert, a ritual for family celebrations. But instead of adding sugar, she added salt to the lemon sauce. It was a recipe she'd known by heart for decades. Her father and sister, Margaret, say Mom is just forgetful. Marissa urges the family to consider something more serious. *"It's just what happens when people get old,"* Margaret rebuts. Her father, who has compensated for years without consciously knowing it, says it is disrespectful for children to find fault in their elders.

No conversation is perfect. All communications are scrambled to a certain extent, caused by the innate and inevitable unique biases we all have where words are concerned.

These biases develop through our individual experiences, personalities, and adeptness with the nuances of language and non-verbal communication. Environmental, interpersonal, and intrapersonal dynamics all conspire to influence communication as well, whether generally or situationally. Not to mention the seemingly wavy line between what *appears* normal and what does not. *Or the degree to which various family members are open to accept that things are different, and difficult, now.*

You need an approach that will help you be brave, caring, and direct in a crucial moment when you must deliver difficult and sensitive information or feedback to another person. In this chapter we will work on applying this approach in the caregiver context.

Even if you never need to have a conversation with someone close to you about cognitive decline – and I certainly hope that is true for you – you might use this approach as a framework for when you have to give anyone constructive criticism or difficult feedback.

5 | THE CONVERSATION

REALISTIC EXPECTATIONS

Some people say, *"Honey, I think you have dementia – please stop driving"* OR *"I think you have Alzheimer's let's move to assisted living"* and their spouse responds, *"Ok, you're right. No time like the present!"* Have you ever met any of those people? Neither have I.

Chances are, The Conversation is not going to go well. Expect that you'll have to have it more than once. It's a scary thing to anticipate. It's easy to postpone. And you're going to be dealing with some relative unknowns when it comes to a loved one's response to this conversation.

Right now, your destination is approximate at best. Heading into totally uncharted territory, we hope to find waterfalls, beaches and rainbows. But the truth is, we might find ourselves in a desert with no oasis.

Although we will not decrease our efforts, we will lower our expectations for this first attempt. Right now we are merely seeking temperate weather. We haven't pinpointed a specific tropical island to visit.

Rather than "winning" the person over to your point of view, the destination for the present moment is simply to open up the topic for exploration as led by our Dementia Caregiver Compass. We can't accurately predict what will happen next but we do know that we can control our own approach and actions.

REALISTIC AIMS

Resist the temptation to debate the signals you've detected. If your loved one responds with *"No I don't!"* when you point out that she asks the same question over and over, your best response would not be *"Yes, you do – you did it just this morning at breakfast"* or *"It happens all the time. I'll point it out next time you do it."*

These statements border on mistakes and corrections. They imply a "you" problem, amplifying that you and I are different. But this is a "we" problem. After all, *if one of you has dementia, both of you are impacted by it*.

5 | THE CONVERSATION

It's worth noting that this is the same approach to take with siblings or a parent who deny your observations. State your observations and allow the opposing family member to respond. Don't disagree with their response. *Offer something more neutral*, like *"We see it differently."*

Marissa will find information from authoritative sources that support her feelings and *share those non-confrontationally* with her siblings. When she finds an article that supports her opinion in a leading medical journal, she will resist the temptation to force on sister Margaret her view as the only view. She will not scribble, *"See, this doctor proves I'm right about the cooking stuff!"* on the photocopy of it before dropping it in the mail to her sister. Instead she will choose *"I thought this article was interesting..."*

People need time to process

Instead of confronting her sister's views head-on, Marissa will make way for Margaret to move forward on the path to understanding and acceptance. Denial is controlled by its owner.

At the end of this conversation, where would you like to be, relationally speaking? Perhaps you hope for acceptance that there is a problem. That might be the ideal objective.

With acceptance, agreement to seek expert opinion comes much more easily. But if not acceptance, acknowledgement that changes are taking place is a worthy objective.

> *Denial is controlled by its owner. Emotionally charged viewpoints take time to evolve; each at their own pace.*

You know best what to expect from your conversation, based on your loved one's personality and your relationship with them. Think ahead about where you want to be at the end of this conversation, what you want the energy between the two of you to be, and what you are willing to let lie by the wayside for the time being.

At a minimum, you will have achieved awareness that your loved one now knows *you* have noticed a change(s). They may think that *you think* they have a problem.

5 | THE CONVERSATION

This is monumental.

Like family photos in a scrapbook – you and your family posing at the famous sites in your travels – The Conversation will become a permanent landmark on the path of your relationship. It will have its own indelible memory, the sort that defines a line between everything before and everything that follows.

Remember that you cannot un-say your words in The Conversation. *Your approach will determine whether this awareness will come between you or, preferably, reinforce the trust you've built over decades.*

This is why I encourage you to first determine your objective, then use the Dementia Caregiver Compass to set your direction. Now you are ready to map the conversation using the following framework.

MAPPING YOUR CONVERSATION

There are six planning considerations, almost equally important to the words you choose – who, when, where, what, how, and why. These are critical logistical matters to plan in advance.

WHO
This is not an "intervention" moment for all members of the family. *This is a conversation to have one on one.* You might wish for moral support "buddy" but the person for whom you have concern will likely feel ganged up on and become defensive right away.

Other family members may also have conversations. That's something you can decide together. But if they do, those should be one on one also.

WHEN
Do not start this conversation when you or your loved one are hungry, tired, or stressed out. *Find a time when neither of you feels rushed.*

WHERE
Choose a location that is comfortable in terms of lighting, temperature, and ambient noise level. *Choose a location that is private.* Choose one where you can stay as long as needed rather

5 | THE CONVERSATION

than one where you might be interrupted after a certain amount of time has passed. It's probably best to choose a location without alcohol, even if alcohol usually isn't a problem for your loved one.

WHAT

What do you say? Of course the substance of your conversation will be very specific and individual, here are some guidelines that apply across the board:

Don't position the warning signs as mistakes. You don't want to come across as judgmental. Avoid the implication that the person is expected to correct the behavior that concerns you.

Similarly, avoid the phrase "medical opinion" – it is too close to the phrase "second opinion" – because it is usually associated with, and in response to, a diagnosis. The phrase *"medical advice" is less ominous* and suggests more of a conversation where all parties are on equal footing.

The word "diagnosis" should be also be avoided. Instead, *get things "checked out"* to understand all the contributing factors to the signals observed.

Keep these language pointers in mind as you gather your words:

SAY THIS, NOT THAT	
INSTEAD OF...	TRY....
"getting a diagnosis"	*"getting things checked out"*
"medical opinion"	*"medical advice"*
"you" messages	*"I"* and *"we"* messages
"you don't understand my point"	*"we see it differently"*
"see, this proves it"	*"I thought this was interesting"*

HOW

Stay neutral. Focus on the facts. You can talk about emotions, but *do so calmly and factually, not emotionally.* Use the journaling process to prepare. Writing your thoughts down forces you to

5 | THE CONVERSATION

really focus on the words you are using and to choose the clearest, most empathetic, supportive, and confident way to express your meaning.

WHY

Even if it seems like "more than just normal aging" *the presence of cognitive impairment does not guarantee the progression of dementia.* Also, the signals you've noticed may be signs of depression or other, treatable disorder(s) or disease(s).

Getting things "checked out" usually means starting with the person's general practitioner, who may see cause for other tests such as hearing tests, vision tests, mobility and strength tests, lab work, psychiatric evaluation, *et cetera. Before any of these tests are performed, diagnosis is premature.*

Still, it may be clear to you that dementia is the problem. If this is the case, communicate with the general practitioner one-on-one, before the visit, about your desires for neurological testing.

Some studies show that hearing loss may be linked to cognitive decline. If dementia is present, vision and hearing tests are recommended so that the person may receive any necessary support with visual and auditory cues.

Give due emphasis to the fact that *it could be a number of things*. Don't pretend you aren't worried about the possibility of cognitive impairment, but don't dwell on it.

Unless you have clinical training, you can only make an educated guess about your loved one's diagnosis. Even if you have relevant credentials, your loved one needs you to be the loving friend or relation who delivers support and comfort. Let a doctor be the one to diagnose. *Let the doctor be the bad guy, outside the family.*

THE CONVERSATION TEMPLATE

Lots of people are unaware of their symptoms. Others are aware but are hiding it because they fear the loss of independence and hope to postpone that. Some will say, *"Well then, you must have a problem too. You just did that yesterday."*

Expect resistance. Expect anger. Expect denial. Expect deflection.
Don't let these responses throw you off and diminish your confidence.

The Conversation Template is a series of five specific talking points to use when you share your concerns with your loved one. After considering all talking points, spelled out below, spend some quiet time journaling in the space provided in this chapter, so that you can think about the words you'll use to fill in each section of the template.

1: I've noticed a change.
Start just this simply. Your intent is to get the person's attention and signal that you're stopping the current activity and changing gears, yet without an elaborate or time consuming buildup.

2: Here's what has changed.
Act like a reporter. Just the facts, ma'am. Be straightforward. Don't provide a long list. *Focus on one or two things you think are most important in making your case.* Compare the new words, actions, or emotions to what you've always observed. It's not that your loved one is "doing it wrong" but something is different, something has changed.

Words like *"that's not what I've come to expect after thirty years"* could be understood as expectations, which are about performance. *Try to avoid words that would imply that the person must simply "try harder" or "do better" because defensiveness may result.*

3: This change concerns me.
Expressing your concern is a show of support. Be sure your concern is on display. But at the same time, try to *express this using "I" messages, not "you" messages.*

Choose words that cannot be misconstrued to mean "what you're doing bothers me." Convey that your concern is related to the person's well-being and quality of life.

4: What this might be is...
Some signals could be symptoms of several different things. You might say... *"You know, these could also be signs of depression or*

5 | THE CONVERSATION

something else. If that's the case and it's treatable, let's go ahead and get some help."

5: Let's look into this. I'll go with you.
More support. Show the person that your loyalty and love remain constant. Remember that it's important to identify and address any treatable conditions. "We are in this together" is the message to convey and reinforce.

YOUR CONVERSATION

Decide how to convey your message ahead of time. Use the space provided on the following pages to write out your initial thoughts for each of the five talking points that make up the template.

Once you've written the words you want to use, try not to deviate. You will choose the words you choose for a reason, so trust yourself.

DRAFT 1

I've noticed a change.

Here's what I've noticed.

I'm concerned and here's why.

What this might be is...

5 | THE CONVERSATION

I think we should check it out. I'll go with you.

After you've have some time to create your five talking points, rehearse it with a friend or family member and get feedback. *If a family member is in denial about the situation, it's best to seek feedback from someone else.* It is important that you choose a person who will support your efforts rather than detract from them.

Ask your rehearsal partner to imagine you are speaking to them directly. Ask them to listen for trouble words and reflect back to you what they heard. Does their comprehension match your intention? The words matter.

Based on the feedback you receive, modify your template in the second draft space provided below. Rehearse with a different partner if one is available. Get more feedback and address any remaining issues before you approach your loved one.

DRAFT 2

I've noticed a change.

Here's what I've noticed.

I'm concerned and here's why.

What this might be is...

5 | THE CONVERSATION

_____

_____

_____

I think we should check it out. I'll go with you.

_____

_____

_____

Have an activity planned for afterwards. You can decide whether you share this plan up front or not. This will give you a good reason to end the conversation if you decide that's necessary at any point. In any case, it will be a way to shift the energy in a different direction.

3-2-1

You've put a lot of time, energy and intention into your preparation. There is only one more tool to pack before moving forward with The Conversation.

THREE

Pause three seconds before responding. This conversation is going to be difficult and fraught with strong emotions, whether anger, fear, sorrow, or some combination of negative emotions. _Give yourself a chance to replace reflexive responses with a more person-centered approach._ Putting space between your loved one's reactions and your response allows you to intentionally convey your meaning in a more effective way.

TWO

Remember that at least **two parts of a person's brain may be dying** if you are noticing the signals of cognitive decline that may suggest dementia is present[i]. If this is what is happening, _the person affected cannot change._

ONE

YOU are the one with "normal" cognitive function – _You are the only one with the power to change your approach_ and to change the situation.

MULTIPLE ATTEMPTS

Don't expect that you will achieve acceptance and agreement to seek advice on your very first venture. Assume you will need to have the conversation more than one time, even to gain acknowledgement. Multiple attempts are normal for The Conversation.

If your first attempt did not lead to agreement to seek a doctor's advice, don't start pointing out "evidence" that you are right. First, complete the field assignment at the end of this chapter to analyze what went well and what didn't, and then plan your next attempt. Second, keep monitoring the changes you've noticed using the gauges in Chapter Three. Third, do what you can to support everyday living and to maintain your emotional connection with your person. Fourth, give it a rest. *Wait a while before revisiting the topic. Give the person in your care an opportunity for self-realization.*

FIELD ASSIGNMENT:

 REFLECTION EXERCISE: Conversation Debrief

If your conversation did not go as well as planned, what are some new things you might try when you attempt the next conversation?

_____
_____
_____
_____
_____
_____
_____
_____

5 | THE CONVERSATION

---

[i] Leonard, W. (2018, November 1). What do you want to know about dementia? *Healthline*. https://www.healthline.com/health/dementia

6

SELF-CARE For CAREGIVERS

6 | SELF-CARE FOR CAREGIVERS

Vivian loves her email and social media. It's the best way to get in touch with her son, George, when he's at work, and to keep up with his grown kids and the world around her. She stays plugged in and checks her Inbox and social feeds several times a day. She's even found some hobby groups online so she can "meet" new people with similar interests. Lately she's getting more email, too. Most of it is junk but she looks anyway, just to be sure. That's how Vivian found out she still had a credit card account with the bank her former employer used. She got an email titled "Update your preferences to opt-out of e-billing" from her credit card company. It had the correct logo and address at the bottom and even a way to unsubscribe so she clicked on the link, hoping she could remember her user name and password. Lately, strange transactions have popped up on her personal card – charges George is now disputing with the bank. An imaginary voice needles him constantly. "What's next, George?" Professional help to watch her while he's at work is not an option right now. He moved in with his mother to care for and protect her. But he feels like he is failing. The constant state of anxiety about all that could go wrong is taking its toll on George's health.

CAREGIVER OVERVIEW

Of the three unpaid caregivers, on average, for each person with dementia, two are living with that person. These are likely a spouse, an adult child, and/or a sibling of the person with dementia. It's logical to theorize that the third caregiver, living elsewhere, is a sibling, another adult child, or a son/daughter-in-law married to an adult child. Grandchildren are commonly involved but not often in a primary caregiving role.

FEMALE CAREGIVERS

On average, two in every three caregivers are women.[i] Innately, women bring some of the best and worst feminine traits into caregiving. On the one hand, women are wired for caregiving and have been since near the dawn of time.

6 | SELF-CARE FOR CAREGIVERS

Anthropologist Margret Mead has been credited with the assertion that the beginning of civilization could be marked by the first known prehistoric evidence of a broken bone that had healed. Her theory was based on an unusual artifact, a human femur dating back 15,000 years.

Mead explained that a broken bone was ordinarily a death sentence in those millennia, and that a human could only survive if the requisite care – setting the bone, protecting, and caring for the vulnerable wounded – was administered throughout the course of rehabilitation. The human of prehistoric ages survived by the ability to hunt for food and escape from, or defend against, predators. Without caregiving, a human with a broken bone could not have been capable of self-preservation and likely would not have lived long enough for the bone to heal.

Thus, Mead connects the healed femur to the earliest known existence of civilization.[ii] A caregiving scenario could only be possible in an organized community, with an established division of collaborative labor and pooled resources to making care and rehabilitation possible.

If we believe this theory, we can extrapolate it to suggest that caregiving is an essential component to, and proof of, civilization as we know it. A female(s) would likely have been the care provider in this scenario, allowing men to fulfill their familial and societal contributions by hunting and gathering food and firewood and defending against predators and enemies.

Part of a sense of self-actualization for women – drive and purpose – is oriented in caregiving. It comes instinctually for women in general and is reinforced by strong social cues.

This instinctual role has its downside too. Their "default mode" may sabotage female caregivers, an innate setting based on internal (and sometimes external) programming such as *"I should..."* and *"I can handle it..."* and *"I'm not doing enough."*

Engrained by thousands of years of social mores, a viewpoint still exists that females who set boundaries for themselves and others are uncooperative, inflexible, or maybe just bitchy. Women internalize these constructs with beliefs that saying "no" is selfish, for example. Consciously or subconsciously, *many women are inclined to attend to their own needs last, after caring for all others, and often only with the "permission" of some inner critic.*

This is not meant as a diatribe on women's social equality. It's meant to examine the ways in which women's inclinations make them uniquely vulnerable to the "occupational hazards" of caregiving. In a chronic high-stress situation that is exacerbated by a tendency to focus too much on others and not enough on self, self-sacrifice can be a dangerous path for caregivers, particularly females.

MALE CAREGIVERS

Male caregivers also have challenges unique to their gender. Society has come to expect that men have the answers or can find them. Males are expected to ward off all threats to existence, yet they are powerless against the progression of dementia.

Male identity is associated with strength. Asking for help is a sign of weakness for many males. And talking about emotions is still off limits in many male friendships. Unlike females, who are more likely to build support networks, *the male caregivers may be more likely to feel isolated in addition to frustration and inadequacy*.

CAREGIVER HEALTH RISKS

These programmed gender roles, combined with the Herculean task of caring for a person living with dementia, make caregivers more likely to suffer stress, exhaustion, depression, disease, and even death during their role as caregiver, when compared to their non-caregiving peers.[iii]

Caregivers who are aware of their own grounding and balance, *paying attention to the physical and emotional messaging their bodies send them, and administering self-care regularly, will have far better outcomes for themselves and the person in their care.* That person cannot enjoy their optimum well-being until you, the caregiver, are experiencing your optimum well-being.

This is why an action plan for Self-Care is a vital part of your way forward. If you aren't of sound health and mental well-being, how can you be your best for the person in your care?

6 | SELF-CARE FOR CAREGIVERS

THE COMPASS APPROACH for SELF-CARE

The **Dementia Caregiver Compass** is useful when we think about self-care for the caregiver. The points of the compass can be applied inwardly, towards self-care, as well as outwardly, towards the person with dementia. *Consider how the Dementia Caregiver Compass might offer an approach to self-care:*

N: NEEDS

Basic human needs that are focused on physical well-being are largely met by lifestyle choices. But what about your own intangible human needs? What about *your* sense of belonging, self-worth, and purpose?

Even as caregiver, your human needs remain intact. Do you feel as if you belong to a community, or do you feel isolated in caregiving? If isolated, is it social isolation? Or, is it a more identity-driven isolation, in that no one understands what you're going through on a daily basis?

At the times when you feel like nothing you try is helping your loved one fulfill their own human needs, do you judge yourself in frustration and silently accuse yourself of incompetence? Dementia is a voracious and unrelenting consumer of caregivers' time, energy and love. *But dementia should not consume your sense of self-worth.*

When something we try doesn't work, we are not failing our loved ones. *We are not failing ourselves. The disease is failing us.* Therefore, we need not stand in self-judgement.

> *You wouldn't be expected to win a game if the rules were always changing.*

It is noble and worthy to get up every day and try once again to make sense of unreasonable – that is to say, unpredictable and ever changing – dynamics without the possibility of rational understanding. You wouldn't be expected to win a game if the rules were always changing. In many ways, dementia is no different. "Winning" needs to be redefined for dementia caregivers.

The concept of *self-worth requires that there is first a sense of self*. Bolstering self-worth means bolstering one's sense of self. In

6 | SELF-CARE FOR CAREGIVERS

addition to caregiving, what other identities do you have? Are these identities aligned with your values and your intentions in life?

Though you will find less and less time for other pursuits as dementia progresses, any identity(s) that feed(s) your sense of self-worth deserve(s) your energy. (We will talk soon about how to protect your time for this identity or activity.)

Fostering these identities is closely connected to a sense of purpose and esteem, which in turn reduces isolation and increases a sense of belonging. You may need to set aside your major personal goals for a while. But *try to keep at least one of your pre-caregiver identities intact.*

Sacrifice is a constant companion on the caregiver's path and the reality is that the other person's needs make urgent demands we cannot ignore. But if we can *see self-care as necessary to fulfill our purpose,* we may help preserve our well-being.

E: EMOTIONS

I talk with my clients about two rules of emotions. In the role of caregiver many thinking, feeling people will keep negative emotions bottled up. They think it's "for the good of everyone" that they stay stoic.

Right? Wrong.

We often have to put emotions in a container to store them away for the time being, planning to experience them later, the same way we put our freshly made chicken and egg salads in plastic containers to carry for a lunch hike – to savor later that day. A caregiver's emotions are often neither tasty nor nutritious but, in caregiving, the sour and unsavory emotions are indulgences we must allow time for too, even if later. The two rules:

1. Let emotions have their life.
What IS good for mental health is acknowledging your emotions and not apologizing for them. We have no control over emotions, nor would we want it. They are too closely tied to survival instincts.

We know that just as there is a connection between emotions and actions, there is a point or line that separates one from the other. *As*

6 | SELF-CARE FOR CAREGIVERS

a caregiver, you will experience sharp emotions, and they will cause you to behave in ways you will be eager to criticize later. You will be short with the person in your care. You will argue unnecessarily. You will *barely* suppress a need to scream. And, if you hear that question one more time? X*%@#&~!

Of course, we try to suppress these urges in the moment. But we can't expect to just send negative emotions away or ignore them until, hopefully, they disappear. We must intentionally wash them from our being in order to avoid unhealthy outcomes later.

Remain conscious of the fact that emotions do not define you. They do not measure your goodness or perceived lack thereof. Knowing this, allow yourself to feel negative emotions fully.

Indulge the emotions created by the caregiver experience to the extent that you can. *Try not to let more than 24 hours escape before addressing powerful negative emotions.* Let them pass through you, whether through journaling, meditation, prayer, or other solitary, contemplative activity.

Yoga, tennis, and running are great equalizers, taking the physicality out of your stress. But in these activities we often are just getting away from the negative emotions, not getting rid of them. *Only in still time can you really face off with your emotions and let them exhaust themselves.* By creating time for this, you will be allowing the possibility to let ebb or transform the negative emotions associated with your unmet needs into positive ones.

Are there certain techniques or even mantras you've used in the past, whether in caregiving or not, that helped you move negative emotions through and behind you? If not, ask yourself how you might develop some physical or mental activities to facilitate this transformation.

As a caregiver, I liked to use mantras because I could employ them any time, to support me when journaling or meditation wasn't possible. One of my mantras was, *"At least two parts of my father's brain are dying, but not mine."* Another was, *"You will have another chance tomorrow."* And a third, *"I am a mere mortal."*

6 | SELF-CARE FOR CAREGIVERS

Your mantras will be individual to you, your values, intentions and challenges. They may and should change over time to remain relevant to your situation as things progress.

2: Unresolved issues need to be laid to rest.

There's a good chance that some of the old patterns and sores not yet laid to rest will crop up again as you process the changes in your relationship to the person you love. *You'll not be able to heal old wounds in the same way you might have hoped or expected if dementia was not interfering.*

For the most part, you'll have to assume both parties' roles in getting closure here. Scientists believe that changes in the brain caused by Alzheimer's (and other dementias) start working years, possibly decades[iv], before symptoms appear on the outside. Consider the possibility that some of these old wounds were influenced by dementia long before your loved ones showed outward signs.

It's clear to me now that my father's "eccentric behavior" in his 50's was the very first sign of FTD. My father had high intelligence, graduate level education, and very strong communication skills. He got along well for a long time. So it was easy for us to mistake his changes in thinking and behavior for a mid-life crisis.

His actions at that time caused a lot of hurt in our family. There was no way these things had a chance of resolving themselves once his dementia had progressed so much that he could no longer hide it, when communications were so challenged because of the changes in his brain.

Had I known then what I know now – about how dementia impacts key cognitive functions long before the signs show, and how his dementia hid from us the funny, silly daddy we had always known to trust and take delight in being with – I might have been able to give new space for the possibility of closure on those wounds. I did not know then, but I can warn you of this pitfall.

If you too have unresolved issues, *examine whether certain parts of those issues may have been influenced by your loved one's changing brain.* by mapping them to the information laid out in Chapter Two and **The Wheel of Cognitive Function and Decline** in Appendix A.

6 | SELF-CARE FOR CAREGIVERS

There may be things that concern you now that are not attributable to cognitive decline. If this is the case, consider help from a qualified therapist as you move forward.

W: WILL

Self-care, in all its forms and definitions, takes time. This is time that you deserve. *And, your loved one deserves that you take the necessary time.* The person with dementia deserves care from *your* happiest and healthiest self. Well-being is the result of self-care.

Administering regular self-care takes extraordinary will. Yet, even if you do have this will, your inclinations to practice self-care are often subordinated by the practical matters that surround attending your loved one. Overcoming barriers to the fulfillment of your own human needs will often seem impossible. *Yet if you can will yourself to think creatively, letting go of limiting beliefs and assumptions, it is possible to see new ways to attend to your self-care and well-being.*

We are programmed to put the needs of others – particularly the meek, ill, and impaired – before our own. It's a path wide enough for only one to pass at a time. That may be the way forward in many acute situations.

But with a chronic illness like dementia, we must cast off the limiting belief that the path is only for one at a time. The path must be made wide enough for two to walk side by side.

> *Letting go of limiting beliefs and assumptions allows you to see new possibilities for attending to self-care.*

Will your imagination to create space in your world for self-care. Will your mind to refuse the voice of your inner critic, who is inclined to interrupt you when you take two hours to hit the gym. Tell that voice that it's not two hours for *you*, it's two hours for *two*.

S: SUPPORT GROUP

For caregiver self-care, the "S" on our compass stands for support. We will talk about getting support from other family members and friends next. "Support" also refers to a support group. More details can be found in Chapter Nine, but don't wait until you reach that chapter to join a support group.

Support groups are free and they meet online or in-person. In a support group, you'll make many needed *connections with other caregivers, who know exactly what you're going through and can offer advice, moral support, and social engagement without judgement.*

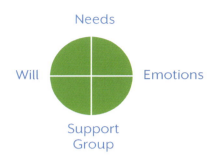

Caregivers often complain of isolation or loneliness due to the fact that it's hard for others to imagine what dementia caregiving is really like, unless they have been close to a person living with dementia. Being close to the caregiver isn't always enough to understand what it's like to walk in those shoes.

Feelings of *isolation and loneliness are not hallmarks of well-being* for caregivers. The support group is a place where you can rant those negative emotions, receive validation, and then feel their grip loosen. That's why joining a support group is a powerful move in self-care. More information about support groups, including how to find one, is provided in Chapter Eleven.

SELF-CARE FOR CAREGIVERS

The plane is going down. Secure your oxygen mask first. It is not possible to be good at caring for a person with dementia if you are not good at taking care of yourself.

Awareness about *your own self-care and well-being* is something you will need to bring with you every step of the way in caregiving. Self-care is focusing your nurturing skills inward.

Self-care means taking an active role in protecting your own well-being and happiness, especially in times of stress.

As you are vigilant about the nutrition, physical activity, social activity, and cognitive activity of the person in your care, so must you be *vigilant with yourself in all areas of your health to stay "fit"* on your caregiving trek.

6 | SELF-CARE FOR CAREGIVERS

You may ask, "Where will I find the time and energy to stay healthy and fit in all these areas?" Good question! If the recommendations that follow seem daunting, it's because you are reasonable and realistic. It's not necessary to follow every one of these recommendations to a tee. Try implementing lifestyle changes gradually, modifying or adding something new each week. You may have to experiment to find what works and will be sustainable for *you*.

Perfection is not the goal and it's unattainable anyway. Instead, go easier on yourself. Just try to find will, power, and ability for self-care today, and exercise it to the extent that you can. When lifestyle choices exist, choose well more often than you choose poorly. Then, leave yesterday's "transgressions" behind and try instead to just focus on this day.

LIFESTYLE FACTORS

Nutritious, balanced diet:

A heart-healthy diet is a brain healthy diet. Focus on eating lots of *good food that appropriately balances good/bad fats and is high in micronutrients and antioxidants*. Also, eat several servings of fresh fruits and vegetables every day including plant-derived proteins.

Regular exercise:

The heart rate should be elevated for sustained periods of time. This exercise should include complex coordinated movement, involving *a multiplicity of different movements for hands and feet*. Ballroom dancing, sports, yoga, and Pilates involve complex coordinated movement.

Running, swimming, cycling and walking are all good forms of regular exercise. Simplistic coordinated exercises such as these offer many health benefits, especially sustained cardio. But repetitive exercise doesn't stimulate the brain in the same way as complex coordinated movement. So *add complex exercise involving coordination that you have to think about consciously* in order to execute successfully.

Although it's not really exercise, *activities that also call on fine motor skills* have a positive impact on brain health. Painting, ceramics, needlework, building models, and playing a musical instrument are some examples of *activities that ideally would be maintained throughout the caregiving journey.*

Cognitive stimulation via learning:

Some believe the best cognitive stimulation is "formal" learning[v], including a classroom, homework, and tests. But the barriers to this kind of activity are high – especially for time-starved dementia caregivers – so perhaps a different criteria for "formal" learning can exist and contribute to your well-being. The point of formal learning, after all, is mastery of new knowledge so that it can be applied in some kind of measurable way (in the absence of other means, determined by you!) through performance evaluation.

Along these lines, "formal" learning for caregivers might be a hobby, if your effort advances your skill level by dedication to actually *learning and using new information you acquire.*

Crossword puzzles and other brain games are fine and should continue if enjoyed. But the emphasis here is on learning new things. Crosswords are fun and they test our knowledge and memory, but they rarely *teach*. Reading is similar. Unless a mastery of the story or material can be demonstrated somehow, as in a written book review or book report for a book club, it's not necessarily *new learning*.

Social engagement:

It's ironic that those living with dementia need social engagement to help them both cognitively and emotionally, yet they often disengage. It's also ironic that the demands of the caregiving role rob family members of their own time and their ordinary routines; *social engagement often hangs in the balance*. Finding a time for social engagement can seem challenging, on top of your role as caregiver. How might you *combine brain healthy activities to be more efficient?*

Perhaps you do join that book club. It will allow you to pair cognitive stimulation (reading and reporting on a book you are assigned) with social time (meeting as a group to talk about your mutual interest in books and the current titles your exploring). Or

6 | SELF-CARE FOR CAREGIVERS

create a golf foursome and socialize as you exercise (provided you're walking the course to get cardio *and* coordinated exercise).

Water:

Water will purge toxins from all of your systems, to benefit joint movement, skin clarity, digestion, and mood. *Six to eight eight-ounce glasses per day* is recommended to gain maximum benefit of hydration for body and brain.

It's not easy to drink this much water, especially on a caregiver's busy schedule. So, if it helps to make water more interesting, and therefore palatable enough to consume in this volume, try flavoring the water with fruit or vegetables like strawberries or cucumbers. There is no real nutritional benefit to these additions, but they may make it easier to drink as much water as is recommended.

Alcohol is dehydrating. For every glass of alcohol you consume, try to drink a full glass of water.[vi] Coffee, tea, and soda are diuretics and should be consumed, like alcohol, in moderation so as not to contradict your hydration efforts.

Spiritual time:

Caregivers benefit from contemplative time. Time to escape. Time to process. Time to build themselves up. It is so easy to be self-critical and pessimistic. Neither is good for mental health. It's helpful to connect with your higher power and/or with your own spirit. Try to make regular time for this, as you do with exercise, learning, and social engagement. The portability of spiritual time makes it perhaps the most accessible/attainable of all these recommendations.

The great thing about spiritual time is that it can be so portable and spontaneous. There is no one right time of day or night for spiritual time, and it doesn't require any specific location or gear. This makes it perhaps the most accessible and attainable of all these recommendations.

Sleep:

Your brain needs time to rest in order to purge toxins every single night and reduce cell inflammation. *Seven to eight hours* is recommended. If you have to make changes elsewhere in your

6 | SELF-CARE FOR CAREGIVERS

schedule or compromise elsewhere in order to get your sleep, try to do so. *Getting the right amount of sleep makes all the other aspects of caregiving easier.* Plus, adequate sleep will help with your mood and boost your immune system.

LIFESTYLE PLANNING TEMPLATE

Reflecting on your present lifestyle, in what ways might you modify lifestyle factors to more optimally support you in your caregiving role? Use Table 6.1, Lifestyle Planning Template, to make any notes about new lifestyle intentions.

TABLE 6.1: LIFESTYLE PLANNING TEMPLATE

LIFESTYLE PLANNING TEMPLATE

LIFESTYLE FACTORS	DETAILS
Diet, Nutrition, Water	Low/healthy fat, sufficient protein, lots of micro-nutrients, antioxidants, 8, 8-oz glasses of water daily

What should I....
- ☐ Start doing
- ☐ Keep doing
- ☐ Stop doing

Regular Exercise	Cardiovascular activity, sustained Complex coordinated movement

What should I....
- ☐ Start doing
- ☐ Keep doing
- ☐ Stop doing

Cognitive Stimulation	Acquiring new knowledge or skill and demonstrating ability to apply knowledge in performance evaluation

What should I....
- ☐ Start doing
- ☐ Keep doing
- ☐ Stop doing

6 | SELF-CARE FOR CAREGIVERS

Social Engagement	Maintain close friendships, continue correspondence, stay connected. **Belong to a support group.**

What should I....
- ☐ Start doing
- ☐ Keep doing
- ☐ Stop doing

Spiritual Time	Connect with your higher power or spirit daily

What should I....
- ☐ Start doing
- ☐ Keep doing
- ☐ Stop doing

Sleep	7- 8 hours per night

What should I....
- ☐ Start doing
- ☐ Keep doing
- ☐ Stop doing

As with the person living with dementia, lifestyle choices are part of the path to well-being for caregivers. When the needs of the caregiver are satisfied and he or she has an abundance of well-being, the caregiving becomes easier.

FIELD ASSIGNMENT:

ASSESSMENT EXERCISE: Complete the Self-Care and Well-Being Assessment found in Appendix C.

The only way to really know whether self-care and well-being are serving you best is to stay attentive to it. **The Caregiver Self-Care and Well-Being Assessment** (found in Appendix C) takes a *detailed look at your current state in six specific self-care aspects of* *well-being – physical, environmental, cognitive, social, value, and spiritual.*

It will take approximately 20 – 30 minutes to complete the assessment and score your results. Although it doesn't have to be completed in one sitting, it's preferable to do so, as you will have a consistent frame of mind with which to work. Use the radar graph and guided action planning space, in the pages that follow, for capturing your insights and ideas about how to address any or all aspects that deserve your attention.

After you take the assessment, it's recommended that you make a brief revisit, more of a gut-check analysis, every so often to ensure your self-care plan is working well.

WELL-BEING GAUGE & SELF CARE ACTION PLAN

After completing the Assessment in Appendix C, *use the blank radar graph, titled "Well-Being Baseline" on page 100, to plot the self-assessment results.* This will create a snapshot of well-being for these aspects individually and as a whole.

Transfer your scores from the last page of the assessment to this baseline gauge as in the example that follows: For each of the six aspects measured, *place a dot on the corner of the ring that corresponds to your score for that aspect.* As marked, the innermost ring is five points and the outermost ring is 30 points. *(Round each individual aspect score up or down to the closest ring number.)*

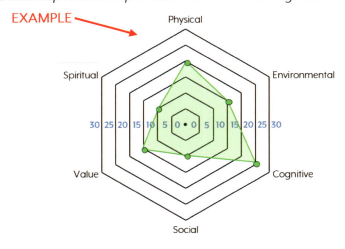

6 | SELF-CARE FOR CAREGIVERS

For example, if you scored 19 on the physical aspect, you would place a dot on the corner, or angle, of the fourth ring from center (20 points) found directly below the "s" in "Physical" and pointing to that aspect. In the example shown, the aspect scores reflected are: Physical (19), Environmental (15), Cognitive (22), Social (12), Value (15), and Spiritual (8).

After placing a dot for each of the six aspects, *connect the dots and shade the area within*. Overall, is the shaded area more or less than 50% of the entire radar graph? If it is less, create an action plan to address the aspect(s) of concern. Space is provided after the blank, baseline radar graph that follows.

The idea is to monitor your progress over time, to increase the wholeness of your SELF, eventually being able to shade the entire radar graph in some future moment.

After taking the assessment, create any necessary action plan. Space for guided action planning is found on the following pages. *Follow the prompts and record the aspect to be addressed, the steps you will take to improve your score(s) for the future, and when you will re-assess how the action plan is working for you.*

YOUR WELL-BEING BASELINE ASPECT SCORES

For convenience, copy your baseline aspect scores from the Self-Care Assessment in Appendix C in the sub-total column below.

ASPECT RATIO	SUB-TOTAL
Physical	
Environmental	
Cognitive	
Social	
Value	
Spirituality	

Reference these sub-totals when plotting your scores on the baseline radar graph that follows.

6 | SELF-CARE FOR CAREGIVERS

WELL-BEING BASELINE   DATE:

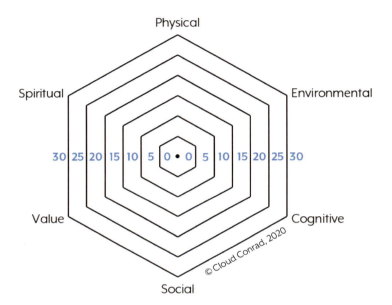

Create an action plan for any aspects that seem to need improvement, using the prompts below:

CAREGIVER ACTION PLAN

Aspect:

Intentions:

Actions/Details:

First Check-In Date:

6 | SELF-CARE FOR CAREGIVERS

ONGOING MAINTENANCE

As a caregiver you are at higher risk of physical, mental, and emotional health problems than your non-caregiving peers. Therefore, schedule time to do "wellness check-ins" at regular intervals to monitor your progress with each aspect of well-being.

These check-ins should be viewed as a very important part of your overall self-care maintenance plan.

As you do the subsequent check-ins, it's not necessary to complete the entire assessment again, unless you desire. You might choose to review the Self-Care Assessment and simply think about each factor and whether you feel that your well-being in that area has improved, stayed the same, or gotten worse.

A series of blank radar graphs follows, as a means to monitor your position relative to your aims for self-care and overall well-being over time. Each is accompanied by a blank action planning template to address any aspects needing special attention.

Plan the intervals with which to monitor your well-being. Write the dates in the spaces provided below in **Table 6.2: Tracking Caregiver Well-Being**, and make calendar reminders to help you follow through with the ongoing maintenance of your self-care plan.

TABLE 6.2: TRACKING CAREGIVER WELL-BEING

TRACKING CAREGIVER WELL-BEING	
Update on	*Update on*
Update on	*Update on*
Update on	*Update on*

6 | SELF-CARE FOR CAREGIVERS

On your first check-in date, use either a newly completed Self-Assessment or your "gut instinct" to plot your scores below.

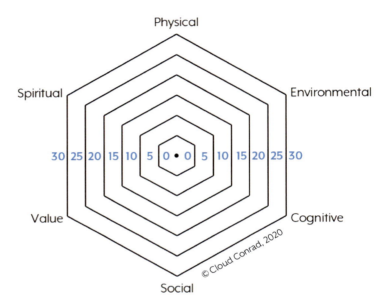

WELL-BEING MAINTENANCE   DATE:

Create an action plan for any aspects that need improvement, below. The Lifestyle Planning Template in Table 6.1 may be helpful.

CAREGIVER ACTION PLAN

Aspect:

Intentions:

Actions/Details:

Next Check-In Date:

6 | SELF-CARE FOR CAREGIVERS

Use this radar graph to define your current location relative to your objectives for self-care.

WELL-BEING MAINTENANCE	DATE:

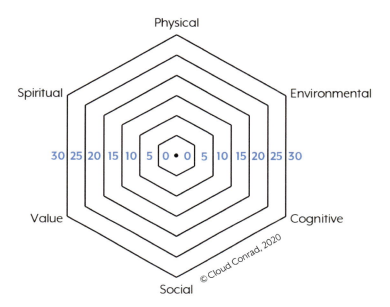

Create an action plan for any aspects that need improvement, below. The Lifestyle Planning Template in Table 6.1 may be helpful.

CAREGIVER ACTION PLAN

Aspect:

Intentions:

Actions/Details:

Next Check-In Date:

6 | SELF-CARE FOR CAREGIVERS

Use this radar graph to define your current location relative to your objectives for self-care.

WELL-BEING MAINTENANCE	DATE:

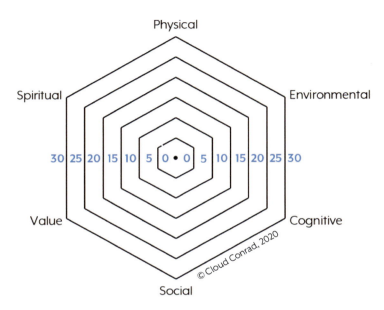

Create an action plan for any aspects that need improvement, below. The Lifestyle Planning Template in Table 6.1 may be helpful.

CAREGIVER ACTION PLAN

Aspect:

Intentions:

Actions/Details:

Next Check-In Date:

6 | SELF-CARE FOR CAREGIVERS

Use this radar graph to define your current location relative to your objectives for self-care.

| WELL-BEING MAINTENANCE | DATE: |

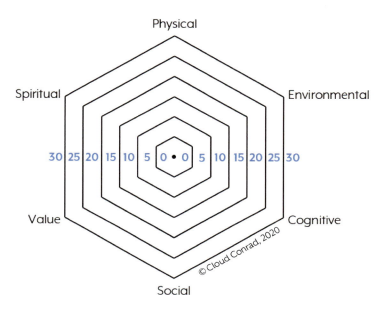

Create an action plan for any aspects that need improvement, below. The Lifestyle Planning Template in Table 6.1 may be helpful.

CAREGIVER ACTION PLAN

Aspect:

Intentions:

Actions/Details:

Next Check-In Date:

6 | SELF-CARE FOR CAREGIVERS

Use this radar graph to define your current location relative to your objectives for self-care.

WELL-BEING MAINTENANCE   DATE:

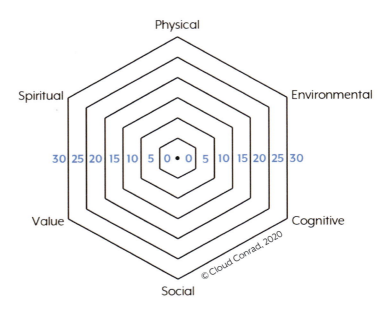

Create an action plan for any aspects that need improvement, below. The Lifestyle Planning Template in Table 6.1 may be helpful.

CAREGIVER ACTION PLAN

Aspect:

Intentions:

Actions/Details:

Next Check-In Date:

6 | SELF-CARE FOR CAREGIVERS

Use this radar graph to define your current location relative to your objectives for self-care.

| WELL-BEING MAINTENANCE | DATE: |

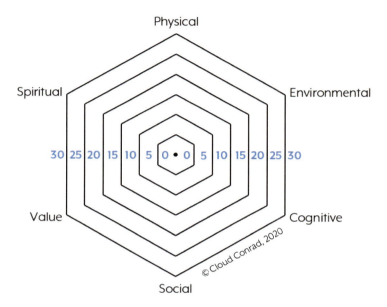

Create an action plan for any aspects that need improvement, below. The Lifestyle Planning Template in Table 6.1 may be helpful.

CAREGIVER ACTION PLAN

Aspect:

Intentions:

Actions/Details:

Next Check-In Date:

6 | SELF-CARE FOR CAREGIVERS

Use this radar graph to define your current location relative to your objectives for self-care.

WELL-BEING MAINTENANCE	DATE:

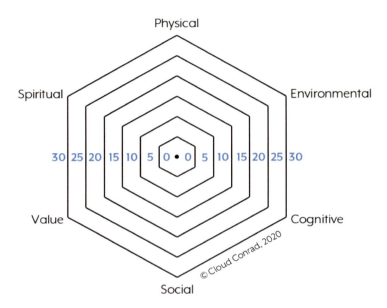

Create an action plan for any aspects that need improvement, below. The Lifestyle Planning Template in Table 6.1 may be helpful.

CAREGIVER ACTION PLAN

Aspect:

Intentions:

Actions/Details:

Next Check-In Date:

6 | SELF-CARE FOR CAREGIVERS

---

[i] Alzheimer's Association. (*2020*). *2020 Alzheimer's disease Facts and Figures* [Report]. https://www.alz.org/media/Documents/alzheimers-facts-and-figures_1.pdf .

[ii] Brand, P. (1980). *Fearfully and Wonderfully Made.* (Zondervan).

[iii] Caregiver health risks

[iv] The Mayo Clinic. "Alzheimer's stages: How the disease progresses". *MayoClinic.* https://www.mayoclinic.org/diseases-conditions/alzheimers-disease/in-depth/alzheimers-stages/art-20048448

[v] Science Daily. (2009, August 12). Formal education lessens impact of Alzheimer's disease -- Even if brain volume is already reduced. *ScienceDaily.* https://www.sciencedaily.com/releases/2009/08/090811161339.htm

[vi] Goins, L. (2010, March 17). How to hold your liquor. *WebMD.* https://www.webmd.com/balance/features/how-to-hold-your-liquor#1

7

NAVIGATING the DEMENTIA CAREGIVER'S ROLE

7 | NAVIGATING the DEMENTIA CAREGIVER'S ROLE

It took Rudy more time than necessary to go to the doctor and back, to Maxine's way of thinking. Dr. Edmunds' office was only a few miles away. *"I guess there was a wait?"* she asked. Rudy arrived home three hours later than expected. *"Huh?"* It didn't make sense to her that he shrugged surprise at her question. While he was off on the far side of the house changing out of his street clothes, Maxine slipped out to the garage, clicked on the ignition, and checked his odometer. Rudy had driven 80 miles! Had he even been to the doctor? Now back, in his sweats, Rudy eased into his chair for the 5 o'clock news. *"Well, what did he say?"* Maxine had wanted to go with him, but Rudy wouldn't hear of it. *"He said everything's fine. Everything's normal."* Maxine knew it couldn't be true. While the newscaster launched the major headlines for the day, she faded off to their bedroom. In the slacks Rudy left draped at the foot of the bed, she found a single piece of paper, tightly folded into eighths. Unfolding the tiny white squares, she saw the scrip, a two word, slightly smeared, decree inked in blue. *"Stop driving."*

Facing a dementia diagnosis is daunting for families. But diagnosis or not, if dementia is present it will progress as all dementias do, causing cognitive decline that is irreversible and ultimately fatal. Until there is a cure, that progression is beyond your control.

But treatable conditions may well be within your control. And if present, they are best addressed as soon as detected.

What is *also* within human control is how the changes to your loved one, your family, and your life are managed. When a family is affected by dementia, they will not be able to manage well without acknowledgement, at least among primary caregivers. *A diagnosis may begin to dissolve any feelings of denial that your loved one may harbor.* Thus, early detection is empowering.

SEEKING MEDICAL ATTENTION

Once you succeed with The Conversation, the next step will be scheduling a doctor's visit. Generally speaking, it's best to start with your loved one's general practitioner, who should initiate a complete physical and laboratory diagnostic course. Do not overlook the possible need for vision and auditory testing as you investigate all potential factors involved.

7 | NAVIGATING the DEMENTIA CAREGIVER'S ROLE

The primary care physician may perform a cognitive evaluation, one of several tests needed to investigate all possible causes of the changes you've noticed. He or she may refer you onward to a geriatrician, neurologist, neuropsychologist or psychologist to perform this test, and others, as appropriate.

Remember that the signals you've identified are not necessarily exclusive to dementia. Remind your loved one of this too. This is why it's advisable to start with his or her regular doctor, who is familiar with the person's medical history and can use or recommend a variety of diagnostics and/or specialists to detect other causes or contributors to the situation.

Simple cognitive tests are usually performed before CT scans, MRIs or PET scans are ordered. These cognitive tests are administered conversationally, without invasive equipment, complex processes, or great expense. The Mini-Mental State Exam (MMSE) is a common test. It can be found online[i] though, which means that it's possible a person can "practice" the test ahead of time. It includes the command to count backwards from 100 by sevens. The Seven Minute Screen (7MS) is also common. In this test people draw the hands of the clock and name as many different animals as possible within a minute.[ii] Another is the Set Test, where people are similarly asked to name colors, animals, fruits and vegetables, and cities and towns. [iii]

These tests are easy to implement and score. And yet doctors don't routinely conduct these tests for seniors to establish a baseline or monitor the results! *Baselines are strongly recommended.* Consider requesting such a test on your next annual exam if you are 65 or older as a proactive measure.

Your physician should also initiate medical and psychological screening for the disorders that may present as memory loss or dementia. These imposters should be ruled out before brain scans are done. Brain scans are costly and inconclusive. Currently there is no *definitive* diagnosis for dementia except by autopsy. If dementia is present, you may receive a more general diagnosis such as "probably dementia, likely of the Alzheimer's (or other) type" but this is certainly actionable.

7 | NAVIGATING the DEMENTIA CAREGIVER'S ROLE

THE ADVANTAGE OF DIAGNOSIS

Since cognitive decline is inevitable with dementia, your loved one is at his or her cognitive peak at this very moment. Now is the optimum time to engage the whole family in planning for the future, while your loved one has the best ability to make thoughtful decisions.

Drugs are available to help ease symptoms of dementia for a period of time. These drugs are widely recognized to be *more effective when administered in the early stages of dementia*, although they don't slow the progression or provide a cure for dementia. *A diagnosis would be prerequisite to seeking a prescription for any drugs.*

Denial may not be limited to the person signaling impairment. Other *family members may also have denial*. A doctor's diagnosis makes it easier to set boundaries designed to protect your loved one, the family, caregivers, and the community. *Let the doctor deliver bad news.*

As soon as you see any resistance wane, schedule a consultation with the primary physician. Schedule these yourself, so that you can be sure of the dates and that you will be available to accompany your loved one to all doctor's appointments. You will have your own questions, and *you want to hear everything the doctor says, first-hand.*

Use this space to list the kinds of tests you think are most appropriate based on your observations. Mention these during the consultation.

Inquire about Possible Diagnostics:

1.
2.
3.
4.
5.

In certain circumstances, a diagnosis may *not* be advantageous. This is an individual family choice. Trust your instincts.

7 | NAVIGATING the DEMENTIA CAREGIVER'S ROLE

STRUCTURE AND INFRASTRUCTURE

To keep you steady and on course, map out a plan for care. As soon as it's clear that cognitive impairment is present, make a family plan. This won't necessarily be easy, but it's important to make sure these difficult conversations happen early, so your loved one can bring their best thinking self to this group task.

THE FAMILY PLAN

One nearly universal fact of caregiving is that most *caregivers believe – erroneously – that they can do it alone.* But to do otherwise, to *enlist a team*, is the only way to adapt to the new world you are facing, in a healthy and functional way.

Ideally all members of the family caregiving team are involved in decisions about each part of the family plan *and* on board with it. **Table 7.1: The Family Plan**, below, includes six components, that are detailed in the pages that follow.

TABLE 7.1: THE FAMILY PLAN

THE FAMILY PLAN

Who besides you?	Statistically, each person with dementia has three primary caregivers on average. You, too, will need and certainly deserve a team of three total caregivers. Who will the other two be? What skills should they begin to develop?
What can continue?	How much continuity can be extended as time passes, by modification of activity?
Until when?	Agree *now* upon when certain activities should be discontinued and why.

7 | NAVIGATING the DEMENTIA CAREGIVER'S ROLE

What's the routine?	Establish a routine. Let the routine be the task master. Every day, make a daily to-do list that includes these three things: • One thing that has to get done • One thing your person wants to do • One thing you want to do.
Personal Fact Sheet	Compile a life history for your loved one that describes their personality, background, and preferences
Life Project	Our human needs for love/belonging, self-esteem, and sense of purpose never subside. Decide on a life project that is legacy-focused and plan how to make it happen.

WHO BESIDES YOU?

There is no shame in asking for help as you navigate the most treacherous journey you will ever endure. Most caregivers will be family members. However there may come a time when professional support is needed. But for now, who, besides you, in your closest circle of family and friends, can take a caregiving role?

There is good reason why you cannot be the sole primary caregiver. And statistically speaking, you will be performing below average if you are caregiving alone. You may think you can handle it by yourself. Perhaps at this moment you are on a solitary journey and doing fine. But this will surely not continue. There will indeed be a time when you no longer can.

At a certain point your loved one can no longer be left alone, safely. Yet you will need to be absent for a variety of reasons – errands, work, self-care routines, and more. Without supervision your loved one with dementia may wander off, start a fire in the kitchen, or find some other endangering activity.

7 | NAVIGATING the DEMENTIA CAREGIVER'S ROLE

Get help now, so that additional caregiver "onboarding" can happen early and as seamlessly as possible and so that you can have the relief that you will need.

Think ahead – who are the most likely and best suited people to join you in primary caregiving? How can they be available? When should they come on board? How will you help them align with your caregiving principles? What kinds of information or training will they need to become informed about caregiving for a person living with dementia? How will you enable them to succeed with person-centered care?

These questions are not ones you can answer alone. Engage family members early and as appropriate in this important piece of family planning. Your primary caregivers should be those you and your loved one agree upon, whether paid or unpaid. Take the steps necessary to enlist your primary team as soon as you can, even if they aren't yet needed on a daily basis.

"Just let me know..." Loved ones, friends and neighbors reliably offer help in moments of crisis. They earnestly offer, Most don't offer specifics – because they can't fathom what these might be – so *we let these vague, yet genuine and generous, offers fall through the cracks.*

How will you summon the courage to ask for help from a willing, trusted, secondary circle? How will you specify your needs so they can be acted upon and fulfilled?

Plan ahead. Identify specific roles or tasks – even if only for now – and make specific requests. As your role becomes more demanding, it will be harder to stay ahead of your needs to give others advance notice when you need help. *Approach them before you need them about the specific contributions that would be most valuable to you.*

This secondary support team is focused on *you*, not the person with dementia. Although they may interact with your loved one, the purpose of everything they do is to support *you*.

What can they do for you? Is it picking up your children or grandchildren from school? Grocery shopping, yard maintenance,

7 | NAVIGATING the DEMENTIA CAREGIVER'S ROLE

visiting with your loved one every Thursday at three o'clock while you go to your weekly yoga class?

What do you need? Write it down. Who can do it for you? When will you ask them?

Make a support plan for anyone who offers help beyond primary caregiving. Use **Table 7.2: Caregiving Team Roster** to help you follow through with setting it up and setting it in motion as soon as tasks are needed.

There is an added benefit to the process of drilling down to actionable items. *Answering the questions above may ease your sense of dependence on others by giving it precise and finite limits.*

TABLE 7.2: CAREGIVING TEAM ROSTER

WHO can help?	HOW can they help?	WHEN can they help?
	Caregiver*	
	Caregiver*	

WHAT CAN CONTINUE?

How much of your loved one's normal routine can continue? How many times can you say "yes!" to the person with dementia? What activities can be modified or supported to maintain as much ability as long as possible? This includes grooming, socializing, contributing to the household chores, exercise, and mental stimulation.

7 | NAVIGATING the DEMENTIA CAREGIVER'S ROLE

UNTIL WHEN?

As a family, how will you decide when certain activities must be curtailed for safety or enjoyment's sake? Some clients have had success by video-taping a brief interview with their loved one, in which the loved one is recorded stating intentions such as *"I know it will be time to give up the car keys when...."* When such difficult conversation needs to happen, their loved one can view the video, see that they agreed to this part of the plan already, and possibly accept the changes more willingly.

ESTABLISH ROUTINES

Routine breeds a sense of comfort and security because routine keeps life familiar. Try to help your loved one feel secure by following an established routine, one you develop together. It will need to change over time as skills diminish but the routine is ALWAYS something you develop together. It's a process that allows everyone to have input and to agree with the final version. Write this routine down. Refer to **The Daily List**, Table 7.3 on the following page, for a summary.

Each morning, make a list together of the things you will do that day. The list should be short but have, at a minimum, three things on it: Something you (plural) must do, something the person with dementia wants to do and something the caregiver wants to do.

We put one thing on the list that needs to get done whether we like it or not. By putting it on the list, we both agree that it will be done today AND that we'll each help the other to get through it. We agree to it because we will both be rewarded for doing this thing that we have to do.

We put one thing on the list for the person living with dementia because that is their reward. This is an activity they choose or you know to be satisfying to them.

We put one thing on the list for ourselves, the caregivers, because it is our reward. It also emphasizes, "We are doing this together." This item can be done with or without your loved one. If they are involved, it will give them a sense of calm to know what to expect. If not involved, this thing is the agreed upon reason why you'll be gone for a bit and someone else will be there for company.

7 | NAVIGATING the DEMENTIA CAREGIVER'S ROLE

TABLE 3: THE DAILY LIST

THE DAILY LIST

Something WE HAVE to do	*We agree to accomplish this, together. Examples might be to shower and shave for a visitor or go to the dentist.*
Something YOU WANT to do	*The special request of your loved one. Many times, their reward for having accomplished the first task.*
Something I WANT to do	*The special request of the caregiver. Many times, your reward for having accomplished the first task. Together, you agree that this activity might mean you'll be away for a bit.*

We add mealtimes and bedtimes, to put a cadence and a cap on the day. Every day varies, but this is what we strive for together.

We make the list in the morning rather than the night before, because the ability to comprehend the future will decline over time. With dementia, it's easier to think about today than tomorrow.

Making the list together promotes a sense of purpose and drive. It also reinforces the overall message that _we_ are in this _together_.

If your loved one attempts to deviate from the plan in a way that cannot be accommodated for whatever reason, or has no recollection of the plan, the list becomes the authority. You may want to keep the list with you for reference if necessary throughout the day. It keeps you from being the bad guy, the one who is in control, who has taken their independence away. *The list you made together becomes the task master.* If it is helpful for both of you to document your collective "approval" of the list by signing it, make that part of the daily ritual.

Even though this is usually a reliable system, it will not always work, because logic does not apply. But the very act of *making a list every morning is comforting to your loved one* because they are involved

7 | NAVIGATING the DEMENTIA CAREGIVER'S ROLE

in the decision making. The task becomes familiar/routine, and they are doing it with you, their trusted ambassador to the world around them.

Think, too, of the people in your community who can help in small ways with big impact. The especially patient bank teller at your local branch, the empathetic grocery cashier who also has a relative with dementia, the barber who knows how to listen to the same story every four weeks and somehow hear something new each time it's told – these are people who put your loved one at ease, reassure them, and help them feel capable in daily living, because they "get" dementia.

If people like this are in your loved one's orbit, try to make them part of the routine. Try to stand in that teller's line, or check out at that cashier's register, or make the appointment with that specific barber. Creating little opportunities for healthy exchanges, outside the closest circle of people, may help your loved one connect with his or her past identity, when peak cognitive function was possible.

PERSONAL FACT SHEET

Since there will be multiple caregivers involved in this journey, it's helpful to establish a personal fact sheet or life history. This document records a variety of information that any caregiver might find useful. This fact sheet includes important information, both practical and personality- and identity- related, such as:

- Spouse, siblings, children (alive and deceased)
- Past experiences, personal and professional
- Preferences, such as hobbies, taste in food, music, and similar information
- Major life moments and achievements
- Medical and legal information, including medical proxy, living will, and/or DNR (using your state's standard form will prevent its being ignored in an urgent situation)
- Power of Attorney specifics
- Life Project details

The more comprehensive the Personal Fact Sheet is, the better. *Feel free to include additional sections. Then make copies for every caregiver on the team.* Also keep one handy, stored in a prominent place, for anyone on the caregiving team as well as for any first responders or medical providers you may need to enlist down the road. If you have a DNR, put it on the refrigerator door, a common place EMS personnel typically seek it.

LIFE PROJECT

Because you've sought medical attention as early as possible, you have the luxury of tapping into your loved one's existing cognitive skill levels to determine a life project. The Life Project, or legacy project,[iv] is designed to create some sort of legacy which your loved one can leave to his or her children and grandchildren, community or beyond. The Life Project calls on the person's interests and talents. *This project is designed to provide a consistent answer to the question, "What is my purpose?"*

The Life Project should have a completion date in the not-too-distant-future. After completed, celebrating this project and reminiscing about it will continue to sustain this sense of personal fulfillment through the middle and late stages of dementia.

The Life Project could be a scrap book, or collage, or a series of recorded interviews with your loved one about major life accomplishments and events. It could be a new achievement which calls upon your loved one's past experiences, interests and given talents, or anything else you can imagine. The best Life Projects are those which:

- are discussed and agreed on together
- have a specific, attainable goal
- can be progressively modified to accommodate changing abilities
- will make a difference, as defined by the person living with dementia

This project is something you both contribute your available skills to complete. *The final "product" should be feasible for your loved one's skill levels at the time it is being created.* Your support will be participatory at first then you'll gradually be facilitating your loved one's activities as their power and abilities diminish.

7 | NAVIGATING the DEMENTIA CAREGIVER'S ROLE

Others can be involved too, to the extent your loved one wants to include them. If this doesn't seem immediately feasible, how might others be involved remotely? How might you use this concept as a springboard for a project more appropriate for your loved one and your current circumstances?

Humans never lose the need for self-actualization. The life project creates and sustains a meaningful sense of purpose, promoting positive feelings like usefulness, engagement, and inspiration.

The Life Project is included on the personal fact sheet so that all caregivers will know about it. Caregivers might be able to use this topic for conversation and perhaps even help to facilitate project-related activity(s) as a trigger for positive emotions.

CONCLUSION

The tools presented in this chapter equip you to step into your caregiving role and initiate your path forward. Keep them with you on your journey.

- The Family Plan
- Caregiver Team Roster
- The Daily List
- Personal Fact Sheet
- Life Project

FIELD ASSIGNMENT:

 ACTIVITY: Medical Appointment Planner

When seeking medical attention, use the space provided on the following pages to make note of doctors to be visited, questions to ask those doctors, and notes about their responses.

7 | NAVIGATING the DEMENTIA CAREGIVER'S ROLE

MEDICAL APPOINTMENT PLANNER

DOCTOR	CONTACT INFO	VISIT DATE

Appointment Details (forms to submit in advance, fasting instructions, etc.)

Appointment Notes

7 | NAVIGATING the DEMENTIA CAREGIVER'S ROLE

7 | NAVIGATING the DEMENTIA CAREGIVER'S ROLE

7 | NAVIGATING the DEMENTIA CAREGIVER'S ROLE

 CAREGIVER TEAM EXERCISE: Personal Fact Sheet

Together with other family caregivers and the person living with dementia, create a Personal Fact Sheet and add as much information as you can think of, including any additional sections that might be helpful. Download a free (MS Word) template that you can modify and complete at *newstreetcompass.com/personal-fact-sheet*.

Post a stationary copy of the Personal Fact Sheet in a prominent spot in the person's home. Make a copy for everyone who will be around the person with dementia including family members, medical and social services personnel, house cleaning technicians, and others who will have routine contact with your loved one. Keep extra copies on hand for unusual circumstances, such as a first responder visit.

---

[i] National Library of Medicine. (Accessed 8-21-2020). Mini Mental Status Exam (MMSE): Tech administered. *National Center for Biotechnology Information*. https://www.ncbi.nlm.nih.gov/projects/gap/cgi-bin/GetPdf.cgi?id=phd001525.1

[ii] National Library of Medicine. (Accessed 8-21-2020). Seven Minute Screen. *National Center for Biotechnology Information*. https://www.ncbi.nlm.nih.gov/pmc/articles/PMC1763549/pdf/v075p00700.pdf

[iii] Isaacs, B. and Akhtar, A.J. (Accessed 8-21-2020). The Set Test: A Rapid Test of Mental Function in Old People. *Age and Ageing (1971) 1, 222*. Department of Geriatric Medicine, Glasgow Royal Infirmary Group of Hospitals http://citeseerx.ist.psu.edu/viewdoc/download?doi=10.1.1.916.2185&rep=rep1&type=pdf

[iv] Rebecca S. Allen PhD (2009) The Legacy Project Intervention to Enhance Meaningful Family Interactions: Case Examples, Clinical Gerontologist, 32:2, 164-176, DOI: 10.1080/07317110802677005

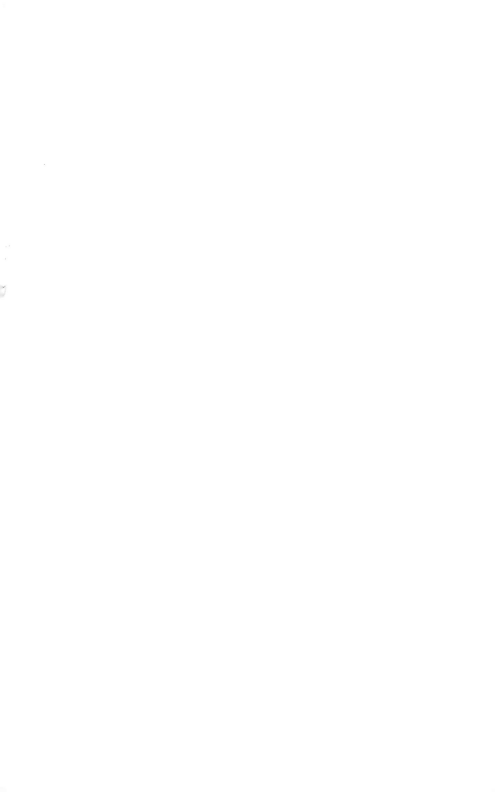

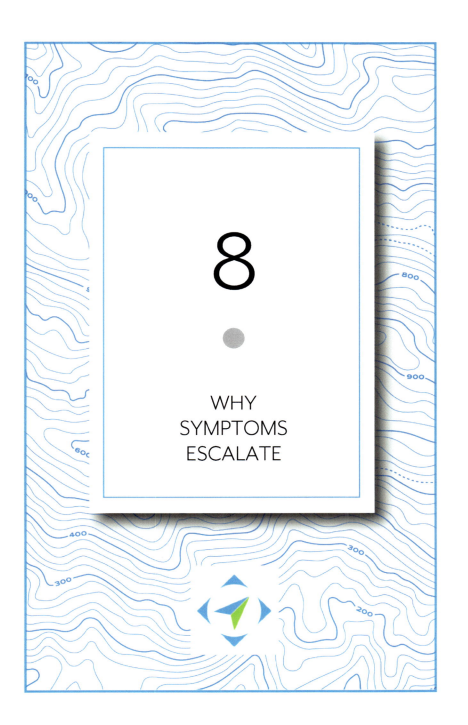

8

WHY SYMPTOMS ESCALATE

8 | WHY SYMPTOMS ESCALATE

For months before Jessica moved her father into assisted living, he complained that the apartment superintendent was using the building master key to enter his apartment and steal his wallet. She had intervened several times to help him buy a new wallet, renew his driver's license and withdraw cash from his ATM, something he could no longer do without assistance. After she'd moved her father she found several thousand dollars while cleaning out his apartment. Forgetting that he had stashed a couple hundred in a coat pocket, or unable find it, he would withdraw more money and hide it in an ever-more-secret spot. The cycle would, of course, repeat. What she'd always known but never proven was that the building super didn't steal any of the dozen wallets she eventually found. When she entered his room this morning on her daily visit, she found him rummaging through his chest of drawers, throwing clothes to the floor as he did so. When he noticed Jessica he turned toward her, shaking the undershirts in his hands at her, yelling *"You stole my wallet! You stole my wallet!"*

Jessica might have responded by arguing back, "*I did not steal your wallet!! Why would I steal your wallet??*" It would certainly be a justified reaction. Jessica was doing everything in her power to keep her father safe and happy, meeting every logistical need she could think of, and spending as much time with her father as her busy life would allow.

When symptoms prevent a person from interpreting and responding to the world around them accurately, situations can easily escalate to create challenging scenarios. *These scenarios rob our interactions of love, patience, and person-centered care.* When we can't understand the root cause of situations that are unpredictable, unsafe, embarrassing, and even inappropriate, we feel incompetent, frustrated, and anxious. The humor in certain situations doesn't prevent such feelings.

The presentation of escalation is as individual as a fingerprint. Various stimuli trigger different responses from person to person and the way symptoms affect those responses is also unique. *But at the core of all escalated situations in dementia caregiving is one central, common theme – unmet needs.*

HUMAN NEED FULFILLMENT MODELS

Where unmet needs exist, humans exert their autonomy and take action based on a motivation to fulfill the unmet need. In the context of dementia, we will examine what shapes the human response to unmet needs and how cognitive impairment creates a divergent path for those living with dementia as compared to their healthy counterparts.

AUTONOMOUS NEED FULFILLMENT

Five basic human needs, as theorized by Abraham Maslow, were examined in Chapter Four: physiological, safety, belonging, esteem and self-actualization. When humans have an unfulfilled need, we respond by attempting to fulfill the need. What ensues is a path of human movement from present to desired state.

However for people with cognitive impairment, the path diverges. The "normal" and divergent paths are described below and delineated visually in *TABLE 8.1: Human Need Fulfillment Models: Healthy and Impaired,* on the following page.

When an unfulfilled need exists, humans imagine a desired state and are motivated to make that desired state a reality – a better present state. Tangible and intangible factors have influence over the outcome.

Will, power, and ability are what determine whether we can overcome and/or harness those factors to reach our desired state. When will, power, and ability function equally, outcomes are predictable, with relative success. We fulfill our unmet need.

THE DIVERGENT PATH

Will, power, and ability are not on equal footing when cognitive impairment exists. Power and ability become subordinate to will. Without power and ability, any actions taken will be disconnected and/or incomplete. Unknown and often unpredictable outcomes are usually the result. *The need remains unfulfilled.*

8 | WHY SYMPTOMS ESCALATE

TABLE 8.1: *HUMAN NEED FULFILLMENT MODELS, HEALTHY AND IMPAIRED*

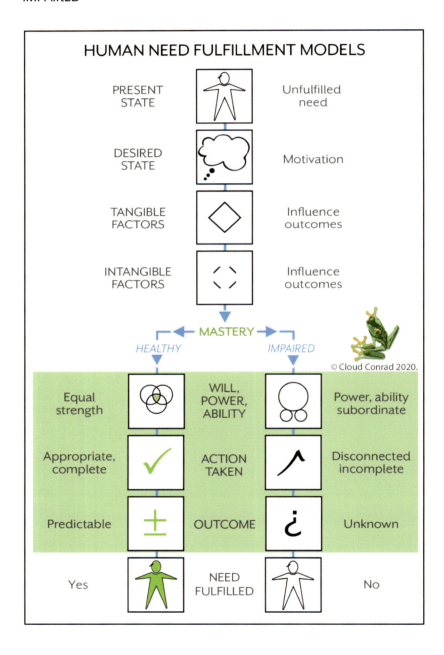

8 | WHY SYMPTOMS ESCALATE

NEEDS

Decades after Maslow initially asserted his Hierarchy of Human Needs, two other behavioral scientists proposed an alternate theory. In 2011, Louis Tay and Ed Dienier published research findings on needs and well-being that articulated a view that human needs existed independently, rather than interdependently, and that there is no prescribed order in which they need to be filled. They also acknowledged that a sixth universal need exists – *mastery* – in support of other scientists' work at the time. [i]

For those living with dementia, mastery (in the green shaded area on the model) is the divergent point on the path to a desired state. In the context of dementia, *mastery ultimately determines whether the need is fulfilled and the desired state achieved*.

With impairment, power and ability cannot be summoned to fulfill a person's need. *However the will for fulfillment remains strong.* The tension in this imbalance leads to anxiety, anger, and frustration. *Inability to fulfill an unmet need presents a perceived threat.* Engaged, the amygdalae infuses need with new urgency but also further challenges power and ability. It becomes a vicious cycle.

This model is useful to emphasize a few points:

- Due to the impairment of cognitive brain function a person living with dementia enjoys very little sense of mastery.
- *In the absence of mastery, all other universal human needs are at risk of being unfulfilled.*
- Yet motivations do not diminish – these are human needs. Caregivers have the knowledge and the ability to be empathetic and supportive when our loved one is attempting to fulfill a basic human need.
- When this model diverges, it is because *the symptoms of dementia impair mastery.*

EMOTIONS

As we saw in Chapter Four, emotions are associated with the fulfillment or deprivation of all needs. These emotions both reflect our well-being and are a product of them.

133

8 | WHY SYMPTOMS ESCALATE

Even tangible needs have emotions associated with them. Why do you think we get "hangry" (when hunger makes us not ourselves)? It's because the negative emotions associated with hunger typically change how we respond in a given situation. These emotional escalations are charted below, in *TABLE 8.2: Unmet Needs and Escalations of Emotion.*

TABLE 8.2: UNMET NEEDS AND ESCALATIONS OF EMOTION

NEED	UNMET NEEDS and ESCALATIONS of EMOTION		
	MILD	MODERATE	EXTREME
Self-Actualization	Inability	Incompetence	Uselessness
Esteem	Dissatisfaction	Inadequacy	Hopelessness
Belonging	Isolation	Invisibility	Abandonment
Safety	Nervousness	Fear	Terror
Physiological	Agitation	Distress	Frenzy

© Cloud Conrad, 2020.

When unmet needs exist, our instinctual physiological response is elevated stress. The brain is washed in cortisol, raising our adrenaline to prepare our bodies for the imminent threat we perceive. *Our amygdalae are in control, intentionally creating a state of physical stress in these moments in order to protect us.*

It is easy to see how our emotions may naturally escalate when needs go unmet. But in the absence of mastery, the person in your care is exceptionally prone to escalation of negative emotions.

WILL

Without power and ability a person living with dementia is aware of, but cannot respond to, threats in the world around them. *Limited ability to see, hear, communicate, perform basic tasks like dressing or dialing a phone number, put the person in danger of failing to cope with ordinary and extraordinary circumstances.*

8 | WHY SYMPTOMS ESCALATE

Yet the will to protect and defend himself or herself remains strong. Therefore the person in your care lives in a chronic elevated state of anxiety. In the hands of the amygdalae, *agitation can easily escalate to a frantic state. Nervousness becomes terror. Isolation or invisibility distorts to abandonment. Dissatisfaction can turn to hopelessness. Incompetence elevates to uselessness.*

SYMPTOMS

Without power and ability, will gets channeled in unexpected ways by these emotions. When situations escalate, it is rooted in the person's attempt to address or communicate their unmet need, an attempt thwarted by dementia. These situations make a rough road and jar any sense of well-being.

Escalated situations are caused by symptoms of cognitive impairment. They are not behaviors "chosen" by the person living with dementia.

COMMUNICATION SHIFTS

In communication, one person forms and articulates his or her message and another person develops his or her own understanding of what that message is. The "comprehension" of *the message received might not quite exactly match the meaning conveyed*, based on several factors.

One key factor is inherent biases which bend our understanding of the meaning of words, whether individually, combined in phrases, or organized sentences. These biases are driven by personality, preferences, and life experiences, among other things.

Context, mood, and regard for the person will also influence message comprehension. Background noise and other environmental and/or physical stressors may also have an influence over how close the message received resembles the one sent.

What was not mentioned in Chapter Two about linguistic skill and communication is how little of it *may* involve the actual words. Based on the work of renowned psychologist Albert Mehrabian, when two people are talking about something ambiguous and it involves feelings and attitudes, words *may be the least important* part of communication[ii]. Mehrabian's research suggests this is particularly true *when non-verbal cues, like vocal sound or facial expression, seem to conflict with the words spoken.*

In such a scenario *the verbal part of communication is considered to contribute only seven percent to message comprehension,* according to Mehrabian. Far more important is the vocal part – the auditory cues processed in the right temporal lobe – the rhythmic, sonic ones. *A little over a third of such communication is vocal modulations like intonation, the rate of speech, and volume.*

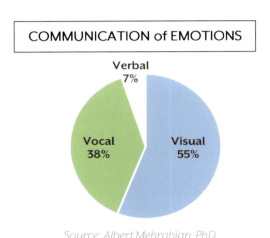

Source: Albert Mehrabian, PhD.

The most important part of communication in this scenario is visual, which accounts for over half of all communication. Our most preferred way to interpret the world around us is through visual cues. It may not be obvious, but it is logical that visual cues dominate, particularly if the sound track doesn't match the visuals.

All of this is accurate in the case of communication between two people who are cognitively healthy. *When a person starts losing vocabulary, speech production, listening comprehension, and short term recall, non-verbal cues will become even more important than before.*

COMMUNICATION AND DEMENTIA

Mehrabian's research in this area is highly specific – ambiguous topics, attitudes and feelings, and incongruent communication cues. This unusual set of parameters makes this research particularly well-suited to the topic of communication when dementia is present.

When things are going fine – the person with dementia feels comfortable and secure, in an environment that is free from distractions – communications may be slightly better than they ordinarily are, for any stage of dementia. But when communication is about an unmet need, the elevated stress associated with that need generates feelings and attitudes that will affect understanding.

Confusion and uncertainty are the underpinnings of this stress – and dementia as a whole, frankly. So ambiguity is inherently present in the communication of unmet needs.

Challenges in visual processing and linguistic abilities brought on by dementia create disconnects between what a person hears and what they see. The person is already likely to misunderstand or misuse words. It is harder to remember what was just said. It is harder to formulate a response. And it is harder to see your lips moving. Given these barriers to communication, it seems extremely likely that the various signals received by a person with dementia would appear to contradict each other.

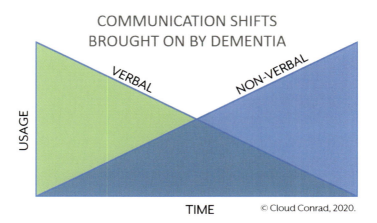

For the person living with dementia, both sides of communication change – how he or she conveys messages and how he or she interprets yours. *As linguistic skills decline, reliance on non-verbal communication increases.* The communication shifts brought on by dementia will mean your loved one will rely even less on verbal cues and more on non-verbal cues over time when compared to someone with no cognitive impairment.

This dynamic can be an advantage or a disadvantage in caregiving. As the vocal and visual aspects of communications gain in importance over the words themselves, how might you prevent the kind of misunderstanding caused by misuse and/or misinterpretation of communication cues?

Mime actions as you speak. Mimic using a fork when you want to signal that it's time to eat, or pretend to shave or brush your hair when it's time for grooming. Use visual data to support the connection between words and their meaning.

Use voice modulation combined with visual cues like facial expression, gesture, and body language to support your message with multiple types of cues, or data, to help prevent misunderstandings.

Be careful though. *Social chit chat relies on non-verbal cues. Your loved one can seem quite capable in these conversations, without getting meaning from them, thus creating misunderstandings.*

Review messages periodically to make sure they are getting through. For example, if the plan is for your loved one to get a haircut at 11:30 today, you might check mid-morning for understanding, without making it a quiz. "What do you think about going to get a haircut before lunch?" (Your person may respond, "Yes – we put it on the list." If so, praise them with something light-hearted like "That's right, we did! At least one of us is tuned in!")

CONCLUSION

All escalations are caused by an unmet need. Unmet needs are physical, environmental, or emotional, but all have emotions associated with them. Unmet needs are closely tied to lack of power and ability in balance to will.

There is often more than one potential cause of escalated situations. But in every case, a person has diminished ability to communicate, accurately interpret the world around them, and adequately respond to preserve their safety and existence.

8 | WHY SYMPTOMS ESCALATE

On some level, awareness about this certainly produces anxiety and sets the stage for escalations. Jessica knows this, so she doesn't argue with her father about the wallet.

Caregivers often encounter escalated situations based on these unmet, or unfulfilled, needs. An understanding of how communication plays into escalations will help caregivers transform negative emotions into positive ones and restore calm.

How to apply a Compass-centered response method is explained in detail in Chapter Nine. We'll learn how Jessica handles her situation, and field test the template with several common escalations, and how to work through them, in Chapter 10.

FIELD ASSIGNMENT:

 CONNECTION EXERCISE: Consider how symptoms of dementia may combine to contribute to escalations.

To prepare for the next chapter, find at least two symptoms on "The Wheel" that, in combination, may explain three situations that you've experienced. Record them in the workspace below.

	Symptom 1	Symptom 2	Symptom 3*
Situation 1			
Situation 2			
Situation 3			

*Optional.

8 | WHY SYMPTOMS ESCALATE

---

[i] Tay, Louis and Diener, Ed. (2011, June 20). Needs and subjective well-being around the world. *Journal of Personality and Social Psychology. (101)*2. 354–365. American Psychological Association. DOI: 10.1037/a0023779
https://academic.udayton.edu/jackbauer/Readings%20595/Tay%20Diener%2011%20needs%20WB%20world%20copy.pdf

[ii] Mehrabian, Albert (1971). Silent Messages (1st ed.). Belmont, CA: Wadsworth. ISBN 0-534-00910-7.
https://en.wikipedia.org/wiki/Albert_Mehrabian accessed 7/6/2020.
This statistic is widely misused but the fact that Mehrabian's work focused on communications about feelings makes this chart, and the research behind it, valid to cite. It reinforces the crucial point that, as dementia advances, communication is less and less about the words themselves, particularly when exchanges are emotionally charged – as is often the case when dementia prevents or impedes the fulfillment of needs.

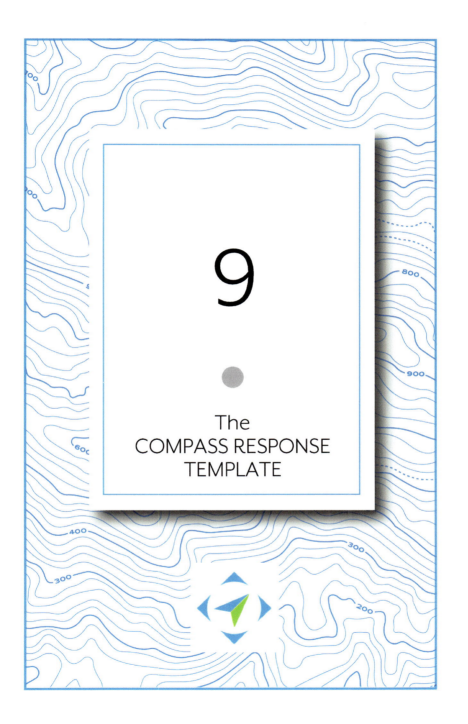

9

The COMPASS RESPONSE TEMPLATE

9 | THE COMPASS RESPONSE TEMPLATE

> For the entire day, Sarah could not figure out what was wrong with Henry. Dementia had mellowed her husband and dampened his lifelong crankiness. On most of her visits he was easy to be around, but not this time. He complained about everything and refused to eat his meals. The nurse who came by to take his vitals was subjected to a list of naughty words that Sarah refused to repeat when she told me the story. Henry wore her down that day, testing her patience in the most incessant way. On the one hand, she felt lucky for all the easy days before this. Yet on the other, her frustration at not knowing how to handle the situation gave way to a nagging fear. She feared that today was the beginning of a new normal. By the time she wheeled Henry back to his room after dinner, Sarah's head throbbed and she couldn't wait to get out of there – just to go home and lie down. So she was not preparing Henry for bed with her usual gentle touch – by the end of this visit she was more focused on finishing tasks than preserving well-being. That did not, of course, go well. Henry wanted to change his own clothes. But in his agitated state he twisted and tugged and soon became tied up in his shirt. Sarah knew to use her breathing to stay calm, but at that moment her technique might have been mistaken for hyperventilation. She crumpled to her knees in despair, uncertain whether to pound her fists against the floor in protest or press her palms together in prayer. And that's when she noticed. She'd been with Henry since mid-morning, but only from this new, low perspective could she see that his shoes were on the wrong feet. She removed them, first left from right then right from left, and then his socks. Henry's tension relaxed for the first time that day. He looked down at his feet. "What a relief those socks are off me!" he burst out, still entwined in his shirt like a straitjacket. "They've been killing me all day!"

Can you relate to Sarah's frustration? The desperation? The fear of a situation out of your control? And then the sense of waste – all that tension endured, all that irritability, over something so simple?

9 | THE COMPASS RESPONSE TEMPLATE

In the midst of a spell of escalation, even when they can understand the cause, it is likely that caregivers will become frustrated and flustered, losing any semblance of the control they have to have over the situation. These escalations can cause tension, stress, and bad feelings, which threaten our emotional or physical well-being. This is normal. You are a *mere mortal.*

Sarah and Henry's situation was caused by pain Henry wasn't able to express, but some escalations just can't be explained. With an effective method to respond, such escalations can often be minimized or deterred. *It takes some sleuthing to examine all the variables and identify what causes escalations, but rewards exist.*

Identifying and fulfilling unmet needs also take time, focus, and patience. And with a dynamic disease, solutions to escalations may work temporarily, and new behaviors will surface even after the old ones were successfully addressed. For many caregivers, this can be one of the most difficult aspects of dementia as the progression advances.

Perhaps escalated situations most brutally reflect the decline our loved one is experiencing and our relationship to him or her. His or her words and actions are often inexplicable – given who the person living with dementia "used to be" – and always vexing, because we can no longer reason with the person to change the dynamic.

It can be so disorienting and disheartening when your relationship to your loved one changes with dementia. It is hard for caregivers to let go of the old relationship and adjust to the new reality that dementia presents.

You are used to the cadences and chords that moved you together for decades in the dance of your relationship. But expecting those cadences and chords to move you in that same coordinated, fluid manner _now_ will trip you up every time.

Instead, try to keep your expectations about your relationship *aligned with your loved one's current abilities.* This will help to protect you both from becoming frustrated and increase the possibility of staying engaged together in happy, healthy moments.

9 | THE COMPASS RESPONSE TEMPLATE

This idea of being *current,* or *contemporary* is important. Dementia is constantly changing your relationship because it is constantly changing your loved one. So "keeping up with dementia" is something caregivers can do to help ward off feelings of anger, fear, loneliness, sorrow, hopelessness, and self-criticism.

Ground your expectations in The Now. As a progressive, degenerative disease, dementia creates a relentless challenge to keep the person with dementia feeling safe, engaged, and happy.

> *"What used to work doesn't work any longer."*

> *"The old challenges are gone but now there are new ones."*

> *"I try and try, but I feel like I just make it worse."*

If caregivers can learn how to stay completely in The Now, they can focus on the certainty that an escalated situation is just for now. That it will subside. That *this wave of "Bad Nows" is a just a phase; it will pass.*

Staying in The Now also allows caregivers to make way for full appreciation of the sweet, funny, joyous, and touching moments that also continue to emerge. *These "Good Nows" hold glimpses of the character and personality you've always loved and admired – too often hidden in the shadow of dementia – and glimpses of your old, familiar relationship.*

Create more "Good Nows" to relish. Keep or create facets of your relationship which allow you to share joy together. Helping your loved one participate *with you* in activities you have both enjoyed doing, and doing together, will make it a little easier to adapt to the new relationship and the new Now. *Make a list of the kinds of activities that can bring parts of the old relationship forward.* Maybe it's listening to music, or cheering on the local baseball team, bird watching, or going to the driving range.

Plan together and adapt your old favorites (or make new ones) so that *the tasks associated with each activity are current with your loved one's abilities.* This will minimize or avoid feelings of frustration and anxiety, which could escalate situations. Be thinking about how you might further adapt and simplify enjoyable activities as the disease progresses.

9 | THE COMPASS RESPONSE TEMPLATE

"Logic does not apply," my mother used to say when we were talking about escalations caused by my stepfather or father's symptoms. Or does it?

Caregivers can use logic and reason in a different way, being alert to the clues around them. These are the markers on the trail that point to the cause of escalation. Only after using the process of elimination to accurately assess the need will you be able to effectively attend to it.

COMPASS RESPONSE TEMPLATE

The **Compass Response Template**[i] shown in Table 9.1 is designed as a systematic method to move through and past escalated situations. Apply the Template to help discover and address the triggers to escalations. Then you can help the person move away from that experience and on to a new, more comforting one.

The Compass Response Template uses a sequence of six actions. It is actually less complicated than it looks, and more intuitive and fluid than it might seem. You're probably doing many or most of these things a lot of the time without awareness of a distinct sequence. It is helpful to apply this template for every escalated situation.

This template works like a flow chart, but without decision or diverging points, moving from top to bottom and left to right, in exactly the same way you are reading this text. As the details are spelled out you'll notice that the process isn't quite as linear as it may seem on paper. You may need to deviate from the Template.

Sometimes you may do two steps at once. Sometimes you may reverse the order of certain steps. Sometimes you won't need to start at the beginning. An extreme example would be that if your loved one was brandishing a kitchen knife, you would start with Step Four, Attend, bypassing any assessment until after the kitchen knife was in someone else's control.

ALIGN

We want everything we do in this moment to be aligned with our bearings. That means we will be led by The Compass. Imagine your spine as north and south and your shoulders as east and west.

9 | THE COMPASS RESPONSE TEMPLATE

Surround yourself with the ideas of Needs, Emotions, Will and Symptoms.

TABLE 9.1: COMPASS RESPONSE TEMPLATE

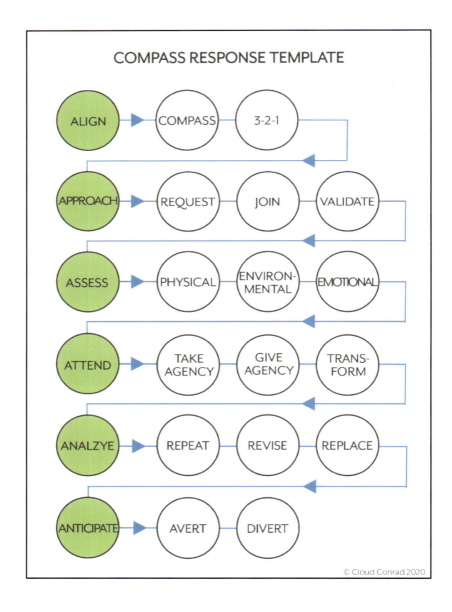

9 | THE COMPASS RESPONSE TEMPLATE

Breathe. Remember 3-2-1. Wait three seconds before you respond. At least two parts of that person's brain are dying. And you are the only one that can change the moment. You can imagine the compass while you wait these three seconds.

APPROACH

No one appreciates an unwelcomed intruder in our personal space. We want to give an invitation, or at the very least permission, before another person comes within three feet of us. In an escalated situation, anxiety is elevated to abnormal levels. *Personal space issues may be exaggerated by perceived threat.*

<u>Request</u> and get permission – do not be the threat. Make eye contact and *get a visual or auditory "okay" before coming closer.*

<u>Join</u> by moving into a body posture that is equal or subordinate to the person with dementia. *Positioning yourself at or below their eye level is best.* When you are at eye level you are equal. When you join equally you reinforce that you understand an unmet need exists and that it's an important one – you can relate. You can empathize.

<u>Validate</u> the person's perspective. *Agree as quickly as possible. Do not debate or correct the person's version of the facts.* Also, equalize your energy level to more closely reflect theirs. Mirroring their disposition bolsters the sense that you are on their side. By validating you assure your loved one of your supportive attitude. This is necessary before making any positive impact in escalations.

ASSESS

Now that we are closer we can get the best view as to which variables might be triggering the escalation. *How might we quickly identify the basic human need not currently met?*

The unmet needs that most commonly spark escalations are categorized, in Table 9.2, as physical, environmental and emotional.

Physical

Physical unmet needs are either related to pain or discomfort. It's important to *address these before looking further – medical attention may be necessary.* Any disorder should be treated right away.

9 | THE COMPASS RESPONSE TEMPLATE

<u>Pain</u> may create visible signs that your loved one has a fever or respiratory ailment, like chills or coughs, but many medical issues are not immediately visible to the caregiver.

Discomfort may be physical (in the person) or environmental (around the person). Discomfort includes things like hunger or exhaustion. They don't mean the person is sick, but they do create stress in the body and therefore call for attention.

TABLE 9.2: COMMON FACTORS FOR ESCALATION

COMMON FACTORS for ESCALATION

PHYSICAL	ENVIRONMENTAL
Hunger/thirst	Lighting
Need to eliminate	Temperature
Constipation	Olfactory
Tired	Noise levels
Trouble breathing	Over-stimulation
Pain (detected or not)	Under-stimulation
Infection	Unwanted touch

EMOTIONAL
Anger
Fear
Sorrow
Isolation
Hopelessness
Frustration
Lack of purpose

Because dementia makes it hard for the brain to detect and express pain, you may have to do a little question-and-answer session to identify physical triggers. Before, you might have been able to say to your loved one, *"You're not acting like yourself. What's up?"* and

9 | THE COMPASS RESPONSE TEMPLATE

receive an accurate answer. But a person with dementia has limited abilities to respond to an open-ended question about ideas (pain) which now may be too abstract to grasp.

Explore this physical realm one question at a time. Rather than, *"What hurts"* try *"Is it a headache?"* If the answer is no, ask *"Is it a tummy ache?"*

Continue with your process of elimination. Cognitively healthy adults can hold three to five chunks of data in working memory at one time[ii] (caveat: *many* variables can affect the different aspects of working memory and this assertion, though widely accepted by researchers, is overly simplistic on its face). If this is true, then five chunks of data is probably overload for a person with dementia. Try to avoid overwhelming your loved one. *If you haven't gotten to the answer in five questions, it's time to move on.*

Environmental

These triggers are often easier to resolve because they are tangible and straightforward. Knowing your loved one as you do, you may be able to realize on your own all of the environmental "too's" – too hot, too cold, too loud, too many people, too busy, too tired, too hungry, too thirsty, too, too, too – that are triggering any given challenge.

Emotional

If your attempts at removing the physical triggers have not immediately changed things for the better, focus on the emotional triggers. Chances are, you'll discover that sorrow, anger, fear, loneliness or lack of purpose are to blame for this situation, alone or in combination.

Imagine it is you who has limited vision, loss of vocabulary, the inability to form new memories, mobility and coordination issues and near-constant dependence on others. You would likely experience some or all of the emotions described above, at least to some degree. Without the capacity to communicate or advocate for yourself, how might that energy and emotion surface?

If you felt anger, how might you show it? What about fear? How might you express a lack of purpose?

9 | THE COMPASS RESPONSE TEMPLATE

But remember, yours are the *projections* of an unimpaired brain. So, whatever you envisioned, this isn't it. Logic does not apply. Emotions, closely tied to will, out-muscle power and ability.

Emotional triggers may be related to the present or the past, or both. Problems in the hippocampus can cause a person with dementia to memory-wander in and out of the tenses. Present day happenings can trigger a past memory or past memories can drift into the present for no apparent reason.

This phenomenon is different from when old reminiscences are used as a crutch for conversation. Some mental meandering is predictable, but other times it can be impossible to anticipate and to avoid the negative emotions they may conjure. You may feel caught off guard.

ATTEND

Attend to physical needs first, seeking medical intervention whenever necessary. *Anything which can be treated should be attended to right away.*

If environmental factors can be modified for comfort, take control. If factors are not in your control, consider other variables you might alter. If the cafeteria is too cold, adding extra layers of clothing or taking meals in your loved one's room might be workable solutions to increase comfort.

If your effort to change the situation and restore balance doesn't quickly change the situation, move on to address the emotions involved. *It is, after all, the emotions of needs that determine well-being.*

In the spirit of the equality created by our shared human needs, caregivers will do well when they attend as an equal to the person in their care. This is to attend to the needs for safety, belonging, feeling valued, and having purpose. Also, attending as an equal preserves dignity and puts retained skills to work.

As caregiver, instead of doing things to the loved one with dementia, do things TOgether. In other words, do with your loved one, not to your loved one. [iii] Practically, it means caregivers approach the person with dementia as their partner – on level terrain rather than

9 | THE COMPASS RESPONSE TEMPLATE

a relationship of dominance and subordination. This means we will need to adjust our movements and speech patterns and energy level to be *with* the person in our care.

Take agency

Initiate the response and attend to the unmet need. Remove triggers. Work in your person's defense. Use language that emphasizes your solidarity.

"I can help with that." "That would bug me too." "You're right, that is a problem, let's go find someone who can change this." If the person living with dementia is highly agitated, you may want to place Give Agency before Take Agency.

Give agency

Ask permission to be involved in the situation and the improvement of it. *"You seem sad. Can you tell me about it?" "You seem lonely. Can I be with you a minute?" "You seem scared. Can I hold your hand?"* Whatever the response, keep The Compass in mind.

Your demeanor, stance, and verbal and non-verbal cues can all be used to reinforce these messages:

- I understand you have an unmet need that is causing distress emotionally, if not physically, and
- We will take care of it together

Transform

Turn negative emotions into positive ones. The goal is always to move the person away from the negative emotions and toward the opposites: calm, confidence, fellowship, happiness, and drive.

By steering your loved one to different environs, changing the lighting, turning on favorite music playlists, or introducing a new activity, you change the stimuli. *When you change the stimuli it is easier to redirect the focus. With new focus comes new emotions.*

So as you move through the building together to find the manager to fix whatever it is that needs to be fixed, and you get farther and farther from where the situation escalated, all the environmental stimuli will have changed. In these new surroundings, the person can more easily be distracted and diverted to a different activity.

Attending requires empathy. Some emotions are easier to understand and find patience for than others. It's easier to identify with your loved one when they are sad rather than angry. It's not always easy to remember the person inside who remains hidden from view much of the time. Respond based on that person – NOT what's happening on the outside,

ANALYZE

This is the time to reflect about the outcomes of our response and *evaluate what worked, what didn't, and what might work better* if it were tweaked next time. We do this in the moment. It's not an exhaustive process like you might use in the business world. It's a simple gut-check to ask three questions:

REPEAT

What worked well?

REVISE

What could work, or work better, with some modifications?

REPLACE

What should I not try again?

ANTICIPATE

Anticipate also calls for reflection. This step is a look forward to imagine which triggers might present themselves and when. To avert this situation in the future, what are all the variables available to me? How might I divert my loved one's attention to begin with?

LETTING GO OF PERFECT

Having detailed this method, a caveat must be included. As dementia progresses, no escalation stays solved. Even if you do everything "perfectly" this time, the disease marches on. There will be more repetitive questions, more hallucinations, and more outbursts.

9 | THE COMPASS RESPONSE TEMPLATE

You can't do everything perfectly anyway. And in a lot of cases it won't be clear what you should have done. There's a good chance your love one won't remember it anyway. So, let go of "perfect" and try to stay completely in the Now. When you do successfully divert, share a favorite joke, or get your favorite ice cream flavor, you can savor every available morsel of joy from a Good Now. And, when things are truly awful, or you escalate by accident, you can stay focused but know that this too, is just for now.

CONCLUSION

With this Template in hand, caregivers can begin to problem solve their individual scenarios of escalation and help restore calm and contentment. In Chapter Ten we'll look at how these sequenced steps can help in twelve different scenarios you will likely encounter.

FIELD ASSIGNMENT:

 JOURNAL EXERCISE: Connect the Compass Response Template to your own experiences.

Capture your thoughts using the guided prompts in the workspace that follows.

Thinking back to your own experiences, list up to five escalated situations which you found most challenging or which came up most frequently.

1.
2.
3.
4.
5.

In what ways might the Template inform your approach to similar situations?

9 | THE COMPASS RESPONSE TEMPLATE

[i] I am aware of several templates or methods to approach the situations that caregivers most want answers to, including those from the Alzheimer's Association community education material and Teepa Snow's Positive Approach to Care ® training material. Each model has merit. The Compass Response Template is a way to problem solve escalated situations that incorporates the principles of the Dementia Caregiver Compass. My own ideas and experiences are combined with creative expression of these other entities' ideas in the Dementia Caregiver Compass.

[ii] Cowan N. (2010). The magical mystery four: How is working memory capacity limited, and why? *Current directions in psychological science, 19*(1), 51–57. https://doi.org/10.1177/0963721409359277

[iii] Snow, T. (2012). *Dementia Caregiver Guide*. Cedar Village Retirement Community.

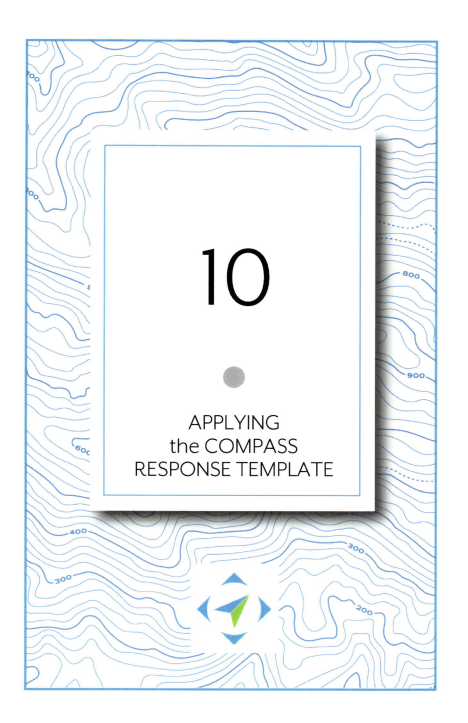

10

APPLYING the COMPASS RESPONSE TEMPLATE

10 | APPLYING THE COMPASS RESPONSE TEMPLATE

> Instead of arguing back *"I did NOT steal your wallet! Why would I do that?"* Jessica says something entirely different. Since her father acknowledged her presence and revealed the trigger for the escalation, Jessica's approach is simply about validation, which she provides immediately. *"Your wallet's missing? That's terrible! Let me help you find it."*

The **Compass Response Template** draws on all of the other building blocks you've learned so far:

- Dementia Caregiver Compass
- Universal Human Needs
- Emotions of Need
- Behavior Models, Healthy and Impaired
- Escalation of Emotions
- Common Factors for Escalation

Now we will see how they can support problem solving using the Compass Response Template, in twelve common symptom-related, escalated situations you may encounter on the path the person in your care takes through the progression of dementia.

When accused of stealing her father's wallet, Jessica might have responded without thinking, to correct the false accusation and refute the very idea that she would even consider such a thing. She might have burst into tears or turned and walked out, hurt by the thought that all her efforts to help him with his wallet were forgotten, unappreciated.

But Jessica understands something about her father that makes other options available to her in response. In the behavior model we outlined in Chapter Eight, we saw a specific point where the sequence of cause and effect diverged for people living with dementia, away from the sequence and resulting outcomes for those with healthy cognitive function.

People living with dementia act on their motivations with an imbalanced mix of will, power, and ability. The person in your care has diminished power and ability to reach their desired state. Yet his

156

10 | APPLYING THE COMPASS RESPONSE TEMPLATE

or her will remains strong, even becoming dominant. *When will is unsupported by power and ability, tension escalates the emotions associated with physiological and safety needs* – anxiety, frustration, and even anger.

In Jessica's scenario it's important that the misplaced wallet represents an unmet physiological and/or safety need even though it is not causing physical pain, discomfort, or threat to existence. Why is this?

There are three things we don't leave home without – our keys, our wallet, and our phone – because they afford us our independence, control, and power to act on various motivations. Without our keys, wallet, and phone we can't pick up the kids from school, replenish the groceries, meet a client for lunch, or anticipate the traffic snarls which might prevent these activities. Over time, these tools become symbols of our independence, control, and power to fulfill all of our human needs – but most basically food, shelter, and clothing.

People living with dementia have some level of awareness, even if subconscious, that they are losing their cognitive function. Therefore their independence, control, and power are at risk. When the tools that support independence, control, and power are not physically present, anger and fear are predictably the primary reactions. These are certainly the emotions we observe in Jessica's father.

His memory lapses are the root cause of this escalation. When he finally reunites with his wallet after misplacing it, he will put it in a "safer" and then "even safer" place each subsequent time. This makes it harder to recover, amplifies negative emotions, and intensifies the downward spiral.

In Assess mode, Jessica understands the real source of her father's accusation is vulnerability and fear, not suspicion. We might expect her to feel hurt, but she knows not to take it personally.

If we were to think about Jessica's situation within the framework of the Compass Response Template, Align is where Jessica has been so far. She has used her compass orientation to identify the real need behind the situation and the emotions associated with it. After pausing to calibrate for three seconds, she is ready to respond to her father's accusation.

10 | APPLYING THE COMPASS RESPONSE TEMPLATE

In this moment, Jessica knows she cannot get her father to accept that his wallet wasn't stolen. Instead of arguing back *"I did NOT steal your wallet! Why would I do that?"* Jessica will respond to the emotions she perceives. Since her father acknowledged her presence and revealed the trigger, Jessica's Approach is focused on **Validate**, which Jessica provides immediately. *"Your wallet's missing? That's terrible! Let me help you find it."* She has not really waited for permission to Attend when she begins to search with him.

Her over-arching purpose in **Give Agency** is to *reinforce the equal relationship* she shares with her father. In attending to the need, she has given agency by phrasing her solution as dual-purpose. She is both offering help and asking permission to give help. When a person already feels threatened by the problems impairment creates, feeling subordinated just reinforces the loss of independence, control, and power.

> *Distraction can be a trustworthy gateway to transformation.*

Jessica is focused on dealing with the emotions of feeling vulnerable and not in control. Her offer to help has already started to weaken her father's negative emotions but she must do more. What if they are unable to locate the wallet together?

Distraction can be a trustworthy underpinning of transformation, if it seems relevant. Jessica says, *"It may take a little while to find your wallet, so let's listen to some music while we look. What about Glenn Miller?"* (It's important to have music at the ready – either for distraction or mere enjoyment – from the favorite genre or era of the person with dementia. Music has a powerfully positive effect on our physiology.)

It's worth noting that Jessica validated her father's perception before she attempted to distract or divert him. In a way, this contributes to the distraction's relevance. Not doing so, disregarding his dilemma and instead offering up some soothing music, would rob some dignity from her father. Jessica can **Give Agency** by letting her father be the one to decide what music they play.

158

10 | APPLYING THE COMPASS RESPONSE TEMPLATE

As they continue to look, the music will change the energy. Jessica might try singing along to begin to create a successful distraction. Between the helping, the music, and the shortened attention span of dementia, Jessica will soon be able to **Transform** the dynamic. Even if they don't find the wallet on the first try, the negative emotions will have been diminished to the point that the escalation will be in the past.

Jessica might initiate a conversation about a solution until they find the wallet, as a way to restore a sense of control. She is further leveraging the technique of giving agency. By participating in the decision about a workable "meantime" fix – the music and the artist – her father can enjoy a better sense of balance between will, power, and ability.

Once positive emotions have been restored Jessica will reflect backward, to Analyze whether she would do the same thing next time or change her approach in any way. Since this response worked, she will try it again if needed. Finally, she will put some thought into how she might Anticipate and possibly avoid a recurrence of this situation.

Misplaced items, especially vital ones like phones, keys, and wallets, are common occurrences. The Compass Response Template equipped Jessica to move through and past the escalation and restore positive emotions and a sense of well-being.

There is no way to anticipate every scenario that will challenge you. Let's explore several of the more common scenarios to learn how the template might allow us to respond in a way that will ensure safety and well-being. We'll apply the knowledge gained from our understanding of cognitive function, the symptoms of decline, the universal human needs we all share, and the emotions associated with them.

In just about every scenario Align, Analyze, and Anticipate will be largely the same. So we will focus in each example on Approach, Assess, and Attend.

REPETITIVE QUESTIONS

Repetitive questions come in different forms. We'll look at three.

10 | APPLYING THE COMPASS RESPONSE TEMPLATE

> *EXAMPLE 1: Harry keeps asking Leslie, "When are we going to the dentist?"*

APPROACH

Harry has engaged his wife Leslie with a question; therefore, he has indicated she is present and invited her to interact. So it's not necessary to complete the **Request** and **Join** steps in the Approach. If Harry seems fairly calm or only mildly anxious rather than agitated, Leslie may choose to **Validate** in the next step, Assess.

If she'd noticed the signs of elevated anxiety, she would Validate and **Attend** right away by answering the question with, *"We'll leave at three. You seem anxious. Would you like to talk about it?"* Leslie focuses on emotions.

ASSESS

Based on your caregiver knowledge, if you were Leslie you might determine information similar to the following, with or without feedback from Harry.

Cognitive skill involved	New memory and learning, abstract comprehension of future tense, detection of pain
Symptoms of decline	Inability to register the answer just given, inability to grasp events in the future, inability to identify or communicate pain
Unmet need	PHYSIOLOGICAL: Possible physical pain or discomfort caused by dental problem SAFETY: Apprehension about dental procedures
Associated emotions	Irritation, anxiety, fear

160

10 | APPLYING THE COMPASS RESPONSE TEMPLATE

Will	Whether Harry wants to go (dental problem) or dreads going (routine cleaning) it is disconcerting to be at the mercy of others

ATTEND

Leslie will **Take Agency** by answering again and again, no matter how many times the question is repeated. If necessary, she'll simplify her answer but she'll consistently try to use the same words. If she can add a visual cue, like writing "3:00 Dentist" on a chalkboard, or white board, or sticky note placed on the refrigerator door, she will do that.

She will **Give Agency** by inviting Harry to express his feelings.

Validate the emotions behind the repetition. Rather than dismiss concerns you may hear, convey your understanding and your interest in trying to help.

They will problem solve together. Is it fear of the hand tools and/or mechanized equipment? Leslie will offer an answer like *"I can be in the room with you if you like."* Or, *"Let's talk to the dentist about what he plans to do today so we can make decisions about it together."* Or, *"You can ask the dentist to numb your mouth, so you won't feel anything."*

These three statements all give agency and help to give Harry some sense of control over the situation, work towards minimizing negative emotions, and restore some balance between will, power, and ability.

> *EXAMPLE 2: Sally's mother Suzanne keeps asking "When is Jane coming to visit?"*

APPROACH

Suzanne seems calm when she asks her daughter this question. Sally can **Validate** in either ASSESS or ATTEND.

161

10 | APPLYING THE COMPASS RESPONSE TEMPLATE

ASSESS

Based on your caregiver knowledge, if you were Sally you might detect information similar to the following, with or without feedback from Suzanne.

Cognitive skill involved	New memory and learning, abstract comprehension of future tense, ability to delay gratification, linguistic ability
Symptoms of decline	Inability to retain new information, inability to understand events in the future, inability to engage in meaningful conversation
Unmet need	BELONGING: Emotional need to connect through communication, fellowship
Associated emotions	Anxious about filling "dead air", lonely in the presence of others
Will	In a state of calm, will does not seem exaggerated

ATTEND

Suzanne is aware of the pending visit, but cannot place it on a future timeline. Sally will **Take Agency** by answering the question again, consistent with the answer she gave last time. *"Jane is coming on Friday."* She will **Give Agency** by adding, *"I've written it down on your calendar. I'm excited to see her, are you?"* Sally might choose to keep the focus on Jane's visit, a positive thing, by saying "We have so much to tell her. Should we make a list of all the important things we want her to know?"

If you were Sally, you would probably have to lead this conversation by mentioning a topic, then asking for agreement from Suzanne whether it should be on the list. *"What about the piano player who came in yesterday – should we tell her he played Moon River?"* This way Suzanne is participating in conversation and also in deciding what they will share with Jane, without actually

10 | APPLYING THE COMPASS RESPONSE TEMPLATE

being asked to remember events of the recent past which, given Suzanne's disability with short-term memory, would be stress-inducing for her.

> EXAMPLE 3: Frank keeps asking his son John, "When is Winnie coming – did she forget about me?"

APPROACH

As in the previous examples, it's not necessary for John to **Request** to **Join** in his approach. John moves closer to his father, who has clued that he is upset, to comfort him. Winnie, his wife and John's mother, passed away less than a year ago; the event precipitated Frank's move to assisted living.

John will **Validate** by meeting Frank's emotional energy level, becoming more somber as he responds with *"I miss Mom too."*

ASSESS

There are multiple triggers in this situation. Frank has been in the assisted living residence for only a few months and is having difficulty learning to find his way around. The unfamiliar environment is unsettling. Frank is resisting socializing with other residents because he lacks confidence in his ability to carry on a conversation, especially with new people.

Amidst the turmoil and adjustment, he longs for the person who he knows best, his life-long love. To Frank, Winnie represents part of the solution, but he also misses her without remembering why.

Based on your caregiver knowledge, if you were John you might detect information similar to the following, with or without feedback from Frank.

Cognitive skill involved	New memory and learning, abstract comprehension of future tense, detecting and responding to threat
Symptoms of decline	Inability to retain new memories, inability to understand events happening in the past, chronic elevated anxiety

163

10 | APPLYING THE COMPASS RESPONSE TEMPLATE

Unmet need	SAFETY: Physical discomfort in unfamiliar surroundings marked by fear and frustration
	BELONGING: Lack of social interaction
Associated emotions	Anxious, lonely, longing for the familiar, feeling forgotten, grief
Will	Will is exaggerated over power and ability

ATTEND

John will **Take Agency** by removing the triggers to Frank's repetitive question. John can't change Frank's living environment. He can't take Frank back to his old home and familiar life. But, he can address the emotional factors affecting Frank's well-being in this situation.

Should John remind Frank that Winnie passed away? Probably not. He will do so only if necessary to avoid outright lying. *"I miss her, too"* allows John a safe way to **Validate** the expression of sorrow because it is certainly a true statement. *Emotions are always true.*

"Remember when Mom ...?" is a useful question to divert Frank's energy away from sorrow by calling on a skill he still has, reminiscing. John is able to change the dynamic without having to change the subject, thereby avoiding the perception of dismissing Frank's feelings.

When you initiate reminiscing activities, choose events that represent major life moments or major family moments for the person in your care. Because of their significance, these memories are more vivid than others. These are often events that took place long prior to when dementia began to reveal itself – when the person was functioning at their peak cognitively.

This is the life the person living with dementia is most familiar with and therefore he or she is a subject matter expert on these events,

164

10 | APPLYING THE COMPASS RESPONSE TEMPLATE

able to speak with authority. When John asks questions Frank has the answers for, he helps improve Frank's sense of control and his balance of will, power and ability. Also when the memories evoke feelings of joy or pride, sorrow will fade more easily.

Engaging in this conversation also helps attend to the emotions of social isolation, like loneliness and abandonment. John can also work to combat physical isolation. If he can draw Frank out of his room, John can help him become more familiar with the surroundings. This might boost his confidence to venture out to the common areas of the facility when John is not visiting.

Frank has always liked playing pool, and this facility has two tables in a quiet room near the cafeteria. John may suggest, *"We haven't played pool in a while. There's a pool room near the cafeteria. We could play a game or two now, and work up an appetite for dinner. What do you say?"*

John has proposed a closed ended question. All Frank has to do is say yes. John will take Frank to the pool tables, and on the way, point out remarkable landmarks in the facility, to support Frank's navigation skills.

Bold colors help people with dementia find specific objects among others. If there are no objects available that had significance in the past, try to find and use brightly colored objects as landmarks. If the person had been an avid birder in the past, the bird cage outside the reading room might be a useful landmark. Or if the person made photography a hobby, the collection of architectural photos opposite the mail cubbies may help build confidence in way-finding, boosting a sense of familiarity with the physical environment.

If Frank can be more confident about finding his way around his new "home" then he may start engaging with other residents. This might further suppress his sense of isolation. John starts making a point to bring his father to more than one location within the facility during each visit, pointing out the landmarks each time for his father. It should be noted that this exercise is meant to build a comfort level with a new place, not teach navigation, which would require the lost skill of forming and accessing new memories.

10 | APPLYING THE COMPASS RESPONSE TEMPLATE

REPETITIVE REMINISCING

People living with dementia enjoy extensive reminiscing about the past. Caregivers hear the same stories over and over. There is often not much of an opportunity to introduce new topics – the person with dementia will quickly revert back to the memory. There is barely even time to interject a relevant comment.

Much of the why's of reminiscing and the reasons to indulge reminiscing can be gleaned from the previous example. However, repetitive reminiscing deserves further exploration because, when initiated by the person in your care, it signals an unmet need exists.

> *EXAMPLE: Phillip wants to tell his daughter a story from his childhood. But Betsy knows this story by heart. In fact she heard it again two days ago. Betsy called today to talk to her father about the upcoming holiday open house at his assisted living residence and her plans to bring Phillip's grandchildren for a visit that day.*

APPROACH

As with other repetitive communication, **Request** and **Join** are bypassed. Since Phillip does not seem anxious, Betsy can **Validate** by mirroring her father's energy and tone – there's nothing she really needs to say to help Phillip feel understood in this situation.

ASSESS

Based on your caregiver knowledge, if you were Betsy you might detect information similar to the following, with or without feedback from Phillip.

Cognitive skill involved	New memory and learning, linguistic ability
Symptoms of decline	Inability to retain new information, inability to engage in meaningful conversation
Unmet need	BELONGING: need for fellowship, connection through communication
Associated emotions	Anxiety about carrying on a conversation, loneliness

166

Will	Will is slightly exaggerated, person is able to compensate in power and ability to some degree

Phillip is participating in conversation the only way he is able to engage these days – by dominating the conversation. It is easy to maintain his train of thought on well-worn tracks. Phillip is the subject matter expert of his memories. He doesn't have to comprehend Betsy's meaning and respond back if he is doing all of the talking. Due to Phillip's loss of linguistic skills related to speech production and listening comprehension, these old, detailed stories are how he compensates in conversation.

ATTEND

Betsy resists the temptation to say, *"You just told me that story the other night."* She does not try to assert her agenda – planning a family visit, over her father's.

Instead, she accepts that her topic will have to wait until the end of this conversation, or she may have to start a new phone conversation later that day or the next that begins with, *"Hi Dad, I only have a minute or two before I have to leave for <next activity> but I wanted to give you a quick call to let you know that...."*

In this second call, note that Betsy does not introduce the normal rhythm of phone conversations by starting with "How are you?" She does not want to invite social chit chat which can easily morph into reminiscing.

By skipping the empty niceties and getting right to the point, Betsy doesn't give her father room to shift the agenda. She has clearly conveyed the limitations of this second call and gets right down to conveying the necessary information.

Trying to steer a reminiscing conversation back to the present tense is often not fruitful. By saving your topic for a separate moment, Betsy has made herself more available to be present in this moment.

Instead of changing the subject, she will lean into it, with encouraging interjections like, *"Tell me more"* or *"I've never heard*

10 | APPLYING THE COMPASS RESPONSE TEMPLATE

that detail before" or *"Wow, you must have felt so <emotion> when that happened!"* The more she does this, the more Phillip may feel the joy of belonging through fellowship and social engagement.

WANDERING

Although wandering often leads to a situation where the person with dementia gets lost, the problem is not always with wayfinding. Wandering is closely tied to survival, as a delusional response to perceived threat. It may or may not be "time travel" – when a person believes the past is the present.

> *EXAMPLE: These days Mary Beth's mother, Ida, dresses every morning in a suit and says she is off to court. Ida has slipped out of the house a few times and has gone as far as the bus stop on their corner before Mary Beth realizes she is not in the house. When Mary Beth finally catches up and calls to her, saying "Mom, what are you doing???" Ida indignantly replies, "I have to feed my family, don't I?"*

It is terrifying when the person in your care wanders off. Unattended, they are extremely vulnerable and can quickly meet danger. Caregivers' adrenaline can quickly spike. After all, these escapes are never expected. The "fight or flight" response in this moment is fight, but fear morphs to anger.

It's easy to respond the way Mary Beth did. She is angry and rightfully so. Ida has exposed herself to potentially grave danger, for no apparent reason. *"What are you doing?"* seems like a reasonable question, after Mary Beth has had to run through the neighborhood in her robe and slippers, looking for her.

The problem is, there is not a logical answer. Ida is delusional, acting on motivations from the past. To Ida's way of thinking, she is not lost. She know exactly where she is going. It is only Mary Beth who feels that Ida was lost. So Mary Beth catches herself and asks nothing more to get an explanation or justification.

APPROACH

Ida has wandered purposefully. *With purposeful wandering, the person with dementia is usually agitated.* Ida has acknowledged that Mary Beth found her, so Mary Beth need only to seek permission before coming within three feet of her mother.

168

10 | APPLYING THE COMPASS RESPONSE TEMPLATE

She is going to **Validate** her mother, hoping to lessen the agitation. *"You're going to work," Mary Beth comprehends.* After showing Ida that she now knows the answer, Mary Beth will reach out for her mother's hand. Permission is granted when her mother reaches back.

ASSESS

Based on your caregiver knowledge, if you were Mary Beth you might detect information similar to the following, with or without feedback from Ida.

Cognitive skill involved	New memory and learning, survival instincts
Symptoms of decline	Confusing the past with the present, delusions promote a sense of urgency
Unmet need	SELF-ACTUALIZATION: lack of purpose, lack of worth, lack of autonomy
Associated emotions	Dissatisfaction, boredom, inadequacy
Will	Will is greatly exaggerated over power and ability

ATTEND

Because will is so great in this situation, Mary Beth chooses to go along with this explanation of providing for her family rather than introduce any counter measures. *"Why don't I drive you?"* she offers. Ida feels safe because Mary Beth understands and supports her need to work. Ida takes Mary Beth's hand and back they go to the house.

When they get home, if Ida is still determined to go to work, Mary Beth will say, "I'll need to get dressed first." But Ida may have lost the urge to go to the office in the span of time it took to get back to the house, the change of scenery and the conversation about unrelated topics that Mary Beth led Ida in as they walked.

10 | APPLYING THE COMPASS RESPONSE TEMPLATE

Mary Beth might further distract her mother before she begins dressing for the day by saying, *"Let's make our list for the day. Come sit by me, and we'll make our plan together."*

Wandering is often related to boredom. Mary Beth has created an activity. The Daily List is a familiar one. Ida has a role in this. If Ida is still able, Mary Beth will ask her to write down the three things they decide to do today.

By the time the list is done Ida may have forgotten or can still be distracted from going to the office today. But if not, Mary Beth will need to look beyond boredom to move past this escalation.

Ida's identity is trapped in the past by dementia. Because Ida will always need to feel a sense of purpose, regardless of her dementia, Mary Beth may call on the past to create a new sense of purpose, tied to the old identity so familiar to Ida. Ida was a court reporter. That's how she provided for Mary Beth and her sisters.

Mary Beth might find an old stenotype machine online or maybe Ida's is up in the attic somewhere. As long as Ida is interested, Mary Beth will facilitate Ida's court reporting identity. Mary Beth will help Ida choose her clothes and get ready for "work" each day. She will help Ida get the machine set up at a makeshift desk in the den. Ida can record family conversations to preserve them, or "practice" her skills watching TV courtroom shows.

It is vital to tailor the activity to the person's skill level or else frustration could escalate. The less able Ida is with the steno machine, the more Mary Beth will focus on the prepping activities, watching courtroom TV and talking about the cases together afterward.[i]

By engaging in the activities that once gave her identity, purpose, and the autonomy to fulfill that purpose, Ida can feel again that she is contributing in a meaningful way to her family. Calling on some of the skills she knows best helps protect Ida's sense of self-worth.

The expectation or goal of producing quality output is not realistic. The goal is to keep the person *occupied* with activities that engage them. It doesn't matter that Ida's shorthand is illegible, as long as she is content writing it. As with Ida's intention of "making a living" *wandering with purpose can often be attributed to a search for the*

10 | APPLYING THE COMPASS RESPONSE TEMPLATE

familiar. A person living with dementia is living in a world that is unfamiliar to them, even if they live at home. People living with dementia are frequently in search of the familiar, which is often their former life.

Caregivers may ask themselves, *"In what ways can I bring the past forward for the person in my care?" Provide visual and auditory stimuli that promote a sense of familiarity in the environment.* Bring several pieces of furniture, souvenirs, and artwork from home when you move a loved one to assisted living. Make several playlists of their favorite music.

For some living with dementia, wandering will be the result of an innocent exit from an unsecured home or building. The person doesn't have a destination in mind, but they wander off and can't find their way back home. *Whether purposeful or not, caregivers should take steps to secure the perimeters of their home so wanderers can't leave unaccompanied.*

DELUSIONS

As with wandering, delusions can be time travels. Sometimes the "destinations" are past events that represented major milestones or accomplishments – scenarios in which the person had independence, control, and power, and used them well. *When you identify the triggers of happy delusions, you may be able to leverage them to help induce those feelings again.*

But other times, the delusions involve unhappy events, memories, or fictional narratives of the present. *Unlike hallucinations, there is a plot or storyline when delusions occur.*

EXAMPLE: When the elevator door dings open on her brother's floor, Jill immediately hears a faint but beautiful singing. As she approaches Stanley's room, the singing becomes louder. Now, standing right outside his door, she can hear the song – "Amazing Grace" – in a lacy, high-pitched voice wafting through the opposite door, ajar, with the "Welcome Sylvia!" balloon tied on the new resident's door knob. Stanley is near tears as Jill crosses his threshold. "They are killing residents here and throwing them down the trash chute! It's <u>horrible</u>! You can hear them scream!"

171

APPROACH

In his delusional state, Stanley is visibly and extremely agitated when he tells Jill this. She will make sure she has permission to come close to Stanley before trying to comfort him. *"Oh dear! I see you're shaking. Can I give you a hug?"*

In this response Jill has also communicated that she understands the problem – Stanley is right to be upset and that she is supportive.

ASSESS

Based on your caregiver knowledge, if you were Jill you might detect information similar to the following, with or without feedback from Stanley.

Cognitive skill involved	Survival
Symptoms of decline	Chronic elevated anxiety, delusions
Unmet Need	SAFETY: When unable to detect and respond to threat adequately, physical and mental well-being are in jeopardy
Associated emotions	Fear, terror, betrayal
Will	Will is greatly exaggerated over power and ability

Delusions are an example of the escalation of fear as a result of feeling out of control and at the mercy of others, particularly when challenged by dementia to interpret and respond to the world as one once did. Unlike psychotic delusions, for most people with dementia the delusion is really an attempt to fill in missing information with imagined details.

Similar to accusations, there's often no one specific to blame in the delusion. The stolen wallet delusion has a specific storyline including "bad guys" identified amorphously, "they" are often the culprit in dementia.

Are there any environmental factors that could be contributing to Stanley's fear? Are there objects or images that remind him of bad memories, or past physical or emotional trauma? If so, Jill will remove them.

ATTEND

It is quite difficult to attend to events that are not actually occurring. It seems much easier to try to assure a person living with dementia by saying, *"No, you're imagining things."*

This will only make it worse. *When caregivers deny the events described to them, they become one of the enemy.* Jill will prioritize **Give Agency** over **Take Agency**. Instead, with her arm around Stanley's shoulder, she will tell him, *"This is scary. Tell me more."*

Play along with the delusions. Jill will nod as she listens and ask for details. She will not ask Stanley why he thinks this is happening or offer up any possible explanations of her own.

Sylvia's singing is symptomatic of the right temporal lobe's compensation for her loss of linguistic ability. But trying to convince Stanley of the truth is fruitless. Logic does not apply.

Since he is not actually in physical danger, Jill will immediately tend to her brother's emotions. By letting him experience his fear through the telling, instead of trying to suppress those feelings, some of the agitation will naturally dissipate.

"When does it happen?" Asking for details suggests the caregiver accepts the person's reality rather than deflect or disregard it. By allowing him to be the subject matter expert, Jill has replaced his fear of being at the mercy of others with having some sense of control. Power and ability become more balanced against will.

As Stanley's agitation is lessened he can be more easily diverted from his delusion. Now Jill can **Take Agency**. If there are triggers she can remove, she will take care of them now that Stanley is a little calmer.

Once inside his room, it only took a few minutes for Jill to realize that her brother was responding to the warbled singing from across the hall. She might introduce her brother to Sylvia – maybe they could start singing together. Stanley may need to be introduced several times in order to understand, and become familiar with, the source of the sounds that disturb him. Another option would be to find out if it is okay for staff to close Sylvia's door when she sings.

What if this doesn't solve the problem? Jill cannot remove the trash chute, but she can talk with the staff and see whether the trash chute can be decorated with pleasing graphics or painted the same color as the wall to disguise it. Maybe Jill and Stanley can paint a sign together that says "Paper and Plastic Only" or similar text to let everyone know that only trash is allowed to go down the chute.

Like many of the escalations explored here, delusions will present in phases. Stanley will have this delusion repeatedly over several weeks or months unless, or maybe in spite of whether, any physical, environmental, or emotional triggers are removed from his environment.

As with all escalations, delusions are at least in part a product of heightened anxiety. Although delusions aren't the result of boredom, keeping the person with dementia engaged with enjoyable and manageable tasks, following a routine that is predictable, and contributing to the ebb and flow of daily life will go a long way toward reducing the anxiety that might fuel delusions.

HALLUCINATIONS

Hallucinations and delusions are similar in the sense that the person with dementia believes that something is happening although it is not. But hallucinations do not have a plot to them.

> *EXAMPLE: Several times a day Elsie starts screaming and crying out, "There are bugs in my chair! They're crawling on me!" as she swats at her arms and legs.*

APPROACH

Elsie is extremely agitated, so her husband Charles will treat his approach with great care. *"Oh no, Elsie! Let me help you!"* he might say to **Request** her attention, ask to **Join**, and **Validate** her – all in

10 | APPLYING THE COMPASS RESPONSE TEMPLATE

one step. Charles does not argue the facts. He comes to her side. It's important to stress that, *in Validation, caregivers should reflect a milder version of their loved one's emotions, so as not to squander their own sense of calm.* Charles wants to reflect urgency, but not panic.

ASSESS

Elsie is very agitated. Efficiently, Charles will Assess and Attend simultaneously.

Based on your caregiver knowledge, if you were Charles you might detect information similar to the following, with or without feedback from Elsie.

Cognitive skill involved	Visual processing, ability to detect pain
Symptoms of decline	Problems detecting form, color, shadow and reflection, unexplained outbursts
Unmet need	PHYSICAL: Safety is threatened when unable to properly interpret visual, auditory and tactile cues Pain, undetected, can create misunderstood sensation
Associated emotions	Anxious, fearful, angry
Will	Will is greatly exaggerated over power and ability

ATTEND

Charles will join Elsie's reality right away, swatting the bugs away with her. Coming to her rescue will help Elsie begin to de-escalate.

Charles will not be able to swat all the bugs away, so he might say, *"Let's move into another room until all of these bugs are gone."* If Elsie

10 | APPLYING THE COMPASS RESPONSE TEMPLATE

were in assisted living, Charles might say, *"We need to get your room treated. But we'll have to leave here for a while when they spray. We can tell the nurses about it when we pass their desk on the way to the elevator."*

By changing the environment, Charles can better determine whether this is a problem with visual processing or a signal of physical pain or discomfort.

If Elsie sees bugs in the next place she is taken, or remains agitated in the new environment, it might suggest that pain from infection or other physical malady is creating odd sensations. If Elsie has an infection, maybe the chills she feels are misinterpreted as bugs. In that scenario, Charles would ask a few questions to try to identify a physical unmet need. If the escalation persists he would order lab tests so as to treat any medical issue immediately.

But if Elsie remains calm in a new environment, it may have been the unexpected play of light that shadows can create. Charles should ask himself whether the bugs appear at the same time of day.

If this is the case, perhaps sunlight is creating problems through the windows. *Drawn blinds and curtains can help reduce troubling shadows and reflections. Also, turning on interior lamps and overhead lights will reduce the presence of shadows.*

The sensation of air moving over the skin – perhaps light wind from an open window or moving air from an HVAC vent – might also be interpreted as bugs crawling over the skin. If this is a possible factor, adjust accordingly.

VIOLENT OUTBURSTS

When a person living with dementia hits, kicks, spits, shoves, or shows other aggression towards a caregiver it may be motivated by pain, strong dislike, or fear.

EXAMPLE: Richard grabbed Lila by her wrist and held it firmly, barking out, "Get away from me with that tourniquet!" before shoving her arm away. Lila had been holding the blood pressure cuff out in front of her as she approached Richard, preparing to take his blood pressure.

10 | APPLYING THE COMPASS RESPONSE TEMPLATE

APPROACH

Lila will back away to a safe distance – far enough so that Richard can't reach her from where he's sitting and far enough so that Richard won't feel so threatened. She sees that he is not ready to permit her inside his personal space, so she grabs the nearest chair and drags it to a place in front of Richard but about eight feet away. Seated in his line of sight, at eye level, Lila begins to **Validate** Richard.

"I must have startled you. I'm sorry." Instead of telling him it isn't a tourniquet, she merely points to it saying, *I was going to take your blood pressure. We usually do it right after lunch."*

Mindful of her body stance, Lila does not raise the blood pressure cuff up when she is explaining to Richard her intention. Instead she keeps it still and uses her other hand to point to it. *If a person is agitated, lifting any object upward, especially quickly, can be perceived as a threat.*

Lila realizes she should have approached Richard from the front at first. If he wasn't aware of her presence she may have created a case of unwanted touch, but because his reaction was so strong, she needs to probe further.

ASSESS

Lila will try to identify any physical triggers which might have intensified Richard's reaction. Instead of asking an abstract question such as *"Do you feel okay?"* Lila will ask Richard a few closed ended questions to narrow down any possible source of pain or discomfort.

"Does your arm hurt?" Richard referred to the pressure cuff as a tourniquet. It might be that he was searching for a word to replace the ones he couldn't find. His word use was either a clever choice or one that reveals a focus on pain. Richard grunts no.

"Do you have a headache?" No.

"Is it heartburn?" Lila asks, pointing to her sternum. Richard nods.

Based on your caregiver knowledge, Lila might detect information similar to that which follows.

10 | APPLYING THE COMPASS RESPONSE TEMPLATE

Cognitive skill involved	Visual processing, ability to detect pain
Symptoms of decline	Limited field of vision, unexplained outbursts
Unmet need	PHYSIOLOGICAL: Pain may be present that cannot be expressed SAFETY : Physical threat is sensed when a person is approached from the side
Associated emotions	Anxious, fearful, anger
Will	Will is greatly exaggerated over power and ability

ATTEND

Lila has already attended to one trigger, her surprise approach, by changing her body relative to Richard's. Now she will need to get him some heartburn relief. When she returns with it she can decide when to revisit him for the blood pressure check.

It should be stated that if the person living with dementia brandishes a knife, pistol, or other object with which the person with dementia could do harm to themselves or others, the sequence would be much different than the Compass Response Template prescribes. *If physical danger exists, call 911 or a facility supervisor right away and separate yourself from the person, while remaining close enough, if possible, to monitor them.*

Do not attempt to get possession of a weapon by yourself. Wait for a first responder to do this. *As caregiver, you must remain safe at all times.*

VERBAL OUTBURSTS

Verbal outbursts can be inconvenient, embarrassing, or hurtful.

10 | APPLYING THE COMPASS RESPONSE TEMPLATE

> EXAMPLE: "Just look at that aide." Patsy points the aide out to her son David as the aide walks by their table. "Somebody ought to tell her those leggings show how big her a** is."

Although inappropriate, verbal outbursts are not intentional. Even if the words used are articulate, they may not express the speaker's true feelings if dementia is involved.

In this case, Patsy displays the lack of empathy, loss of inhibition, and/or loss of self-control that has developed with dementia's progression. The use of naughty words signals that she has limited access to her "good words' these days.

APPROACH

Because David is seated at a table with Patsy, in the cafeteria of her nursing home, there is no need to **Request** or **Join**. There is not a need or emotion to **Validate** either. But, instead of correcting her or expressing any disapproval, David will move right to Assess.

ASSESS

Patsy was more reserved in her pre-dementia days. She would not have even commented on the aide's leggings, let alone criticize or speak loudly enough to be heard by the aide.

Based on your caregiver knowledge, if you were David you might detect information similar to the following.

Cognitive skill involved	Linguistic skills, inhibition
Symptoms of decline	Inappropriate language, lack of self-control, lack of empathy
Unmet need	PHYSIOLOGICAL: Physical pain may be present that cannot be expressed BELONGING: Need for fellowship yet unable to converse as before
Associated emotions	Irritated, frustrated, lonely

10 | APPLYING THE COMPASS RESPONSE TEMPLATE

Will	Will is exaggerated over power and ability

David wonders if Patsy's fever is back. She had a urinary tract infection, but she finished a round of antibiotics just a few days ago. He feels her forehead to see if she has a temperature. He takes her hand to see if her palm is cool, as it normally is, or clammy. She seems okay, but just to be sure he asks, *"Mom, did your urinary tract infection come back? Does it hurt when you tinkle?"*

For some, this might be too sophisticated a question. But Patsy understands the yes-or-no question, at least the second one, and shakes her head no. She doesn't seem agitated or uncomfortable. David considers the possibility of discomfort. Patsy's night aide noted in the caregiver journal that Patsy had not slept well the prior two nights. Perhaps she is tired. David decides to see if she will take a nap when they get back to the room.

If Patsy's not reacting to an unmet physiological need, then what might be happening emotionally? Her inappropriate language is likely the product of lost executive skill. Lack of empathy and lack of inhibition seem to be contributing to these escalations.

Patsy is trying to make conversation with her son while he visits. But she can't really participate in conversation, so social chit chat with some bad words sprinkled in is what she relies on more often these days – her skills in the right temporal lobe are still strong and able to compensate.

The emotional trigger is the loneliness and isolation she feels, even in the presence of others. These feelings are caused by her inability to participate in interesting conversations anymore.

ATTEND

In the meantime, here comes the aide in leggings again. Quickly, David asks Patsy about a topic on which she is a subject matter expert, old *Bonanza* reruns. *"Mom, when Bonanza was on TV, did you ever have a crush on any of the Cartwright boys?"*

Asking a person with dementia about something from the past is not advisable in certain situations, but in this case David has asked

Patsy about a topic she is very familiar with, one from her best cognitive life that's still shown on cable networks today. Also, note that David didn't ask her to recall a fact. He asked her about a feeling and in a yes-or-no question format.

David does this to get Patsy thinking about something interesting to distract her from the aide's appearance the second time she walks by their table. Believing that she was trying to initiate a conversation, he called upon one of the tried and true topics that engage Patsy.

As caregiver, *try to identify "safe" topics and questions that you can use to help the person with dementia feel connected socially. Such topics do double duty, by helping you distract* attention from various triggers that cause escalations. Good news: only two or three are necessary, because you can use them over and over and they will distract successfully many times. When you find good ones, add them to the Personal Fact Sheet to help your fellow caregivers.

INAPPROPRIATE ACTS

Unwanted sexual advances, lewd words, and public nudity are examples of inappropriate acts you may observe from someone living with dementia. Because such acts are not only offensive but potentially illegal, caregivers will address escalations differently than other situations created by the symptoms of advancing dementia.

Generally, **Approach, Assess** and **Attend** are happening simultaneously in these situations in order to protect others. But caregivers have another consideration. The dignity of the person in your care is perhaps most vulnerable in these situations.

> *EXAMPLE: Herb roams the halls of his assisted living facility in the evenings. Sometimes he's in his pajamas but other times he's naked. Tonight, when the elevator doors opened on her father's floor, Catherine finds him walking down the hallway toward her, in all his glory.*

This is a tenuous moment for Catherine. Fortunately, no one is around and it's possible that she is the first person he has seen while out in public unclothed.

As humans, criticism often strips our armor. When we are exposed to it we feel some degree of nakedness, certainly. *But we are never more vulnerable than when we are criticized while not actually wearing any clothes.*

Of course, we are not talking about aesthetics or endowment or lack thereof. The archetypal nightmare about being naked in school isn't about physique. In that dream, our anxiety seems to be about simply being exposed. It's about feeling generally vulnerable.

APPROACH

As always, the Approach has a lot to do with our success in working past escalations. Catherine is fortunate that she and her father appear to be alone. So her job is easier than if she'd been waiting for the elevator in the busy first floor lobby to find her father behind the doors when they open.

"Dad!" she will say, as if greeting him fully clothed. *'I'm glad I found you!"* This is certainly true!

Since they are approaching each other in a hallway, it's safe to say Catherine is in his field of vision. Herb does not seem agitated when he waves to her. There is no apparent physical or emotional unmet need.

ASSESS

You know, based on your caregiver knowledge, that this escalation is not due to lewd intentions, but rather symptom-related behaviors. If you were Catherine, you might detect information similar to the following.

Cognitive skill involved	Self-awareness, sense of time and place, task sequencing, fine motor skills
Symptoms of decline	Lack of inhibition, losing the line between public and private spaces, lack of empathy, inability to fasten clothes

	PHYSIOLOGICAL: Discomfort using fine motor skills
Unmet need	BELONGING: Lack of social engagement, and connection
	Innocent nudity may not be associated with any unmet need
Associated emotions	Lonely, bored
Will	Will and power dominate ability

ATTEND

Catherine will not ask why he's not wearing any clothes. Every second is focused on getting Herb out of public view. *"Can we go back to your apartment right away? I really need to use your bathroom."*

OR

"I'm so glad I found you here. I need to use your telephone to call the babysitter. My cell battery is dead. Can we go back to your room for a minute?"

Whether real or manufactured, create a real urgency to get back to your loved one's room as quickly as possible. Make this urgency about something that's happening to you. Knowing that Catherine is the subject matter expert on her own life, Herb is less likely to resist Catherine's request. She will make some chit chat on the way to his room to distract him from her fabricated reason to get there quickly. Once there, she can simply say, *"Let's get dressed for bed. Then we can watch some TV."*

Catherine helps her father put on his pajamas. While doing so she tries to determine whether declining manual dexterity prevents buttoning pajama tops or tying pajama bottom waistbands. If so, she'll find him elastic pull-on pajamas for easier dressing.

This may be a sequencing problem originating from the prefrontal cortex. It is possible Herb doesn't know where the pajamas are kept, or because they are not visible, he forgets to put them on

10 | APPLYING THE COMPASS RESPONSE TEMPLATE

when he takes off his day clothes. Catherine might request that a staff member set her father's pajamas out on the bed each night to overcome potential sequencing problems.

Also, Catherine will see whether his social engagement can be increased during the day. If a busier day will make him more tired after dinner, Herb may be less likely to stay active at night and more prone to settle in to a chair or bed to be read to or watch television.

The role of inhibition, also from the prefrontal cortex, is to keep us from embarrassing ourselves. Herb may not be aware that he's nude or he may not realize that he's doing anything strange. Catherine really has nothing to gain from pointing out his nudity to her father.

Freedom from inhibition will also invite lewd comments from a person living with dementia. Unlike public nudity, *lewd comments are also abetted by a lack of empathy,* which comes from the prefrontal cortex as well. Therefore those making such comments won't understand why their comments are offensive to others.

Lewd comments may also be the fault of the right temporal lobe. Unable to carry on in conversation as they once could, a person's right temporal lobe will try to fill in the blanks with poetry, prayer, song, profanity, and repetitive phrases. *Lewd comments are often repetitive or go-to phrases used when more appropriate language cannot be found.* Lewd comments are an attempt to connect.

Catherine finds that Herb can often be redirected from lewd comments by engaging him in conversations about tried-and-true topics he's interested in and/or knowledgeable, like reminiscences of the past. *When social engagement is high and people can converse on familiar topics, lewd comments are likely to subside.*

Many people living with dementia will want to act on sexual urges. Natural for humans, sexual urges should not be shunned. Rather, the caregiver should seek ways to *facilitate the loved one's safe and private indulgence in a healthy manner* and without judgement. It's important to stress that sexual activities with caregivers, staff, or other residents are not appropriate. A fellow resident may not be able to meaningfully consent or decline, and neither may understand the responses of the other. Unprotected sex is also a

10 | APPLYING THE COMPASS RESPONSE TEMPLATE

big concern. Where consensual sex with a spouse or partner is not applicable or possible, private masturbation is an option that will allow safe and healthy expression without offending others or putting them at physical risk.

RUMMAGING

When a person with dementia rummages in drawers or closets, it usually signals anxiety about a misplaced item. The longer the item goes unfound, the more the anxiety escalates. In this emotional state, it will become harder and harder for a person to locate the item. It's possible that the person will look right at the "missing" object without recognizing it.

Thinking back to Jessica and her father, his anxiety continued to build as he searched unsuccessfully for his wallet to the point that he accused his own daughter of stealing it.

APPROACH

As Jessica did with her father, we can combine **Request, Join** and **Validate** in one quick sentence so that we can start helping the person find the missing item as quickly as possible. If Jessica did not already know what he was looking for she might say, *"Hi, Dad. Is something missing? I'll help you look."*

ASSESS

Jessica already knows a few things about rummaging and her father's situation.

Cognitive skill involved	New memories, executive function, sensing threat
Symptoms of decline	Misplacing objects, inability to start, sequence, and stop tasks, sense of urgency, inability to move on
Unmet need	SAFETY: perceived risk without an object deemed "essential"
Associated emotions	Anxious, fearful, bored, over-stimulated

10 | APPLYING THE COMPASS RESPONSE TEMPLATE

Will	Will is exaggerated over power and ability

ATTEND

Without intervention, frenzy builds. A person will quickly become angry or terrified. *For all repetitive behaviors, offer to help the person with what they are trying to do.* Start talking about the missing item.

"What does it look like?" "When did you have it last?" "What was in your wallet?" "Did you have any pictures in your wallet?" "Which ones?"

Ask these questions slowly and calmly, or it might feel like an interrogation. Try to break up the questions with comments. *"Oh, that's one of my favorite pictures of Mom."*

Find any means to get the person to start talking, and thinking, about something else. *"I remember when she bought that dress. She was worried it cost too much, but she looked so great in it."*

After a little while, when her father's anxiety has reduced to the point he can talk, she will say, *"Remembering that dress makes me want to look at more pictures of her. Let's take a quick break to look at some more pictures of her. I have some on my phone."*

As a person's dementia progresses, they will misplace important things. The "safe place" Jessica's father put his wallet was forgotten. As caregiver, are there ways you can prevent your loved one from misplacing things, or ways that you can more easily find them if they go missing?

If important items are brightly colored, they will be easier to locate. Also, fetching devices can be attached to wallets, keys, and other items in order to locate them with an app on your phone.

REPETITIVE ACTIONS

Pacing, fidgeting, and other repetitive tasks can signal over or under-stimulation. The person with dementia may resort to repetitive actions when they are bored or when they are faced with too much visual, auditory, or tactile information.

10 | APPLYING THE COMPASS RESPONSE TEMPLATE

With pacing, a person may instead be attempting to move away from pain or discomfort. Fidgeting may also be triggered by being asked to perform overly complicated tasks which they can no longer start, stop or sequence.

> EXAMPLE: Fred paces the hall outside his door, muttering under his breath.

APPROACH

Fred's sister Jenny finds him pacing when she comes to visit him. She will use a calm approach, simply stating his name. What Jenny says next depends on Fred's level of agitation.

If Fred were calm, she might say *"I see you're walking back and forth. It's a beautiful day outside. Will you come walk with me in the courtyard?"*

But Fred is agitated. So Jenny will gently call *"Fred"* to get his attention. While reaching out her hand to him, she will say, *"Fred, you look distressed. Is something wrong?"* Jenny has shown she's supportive of Fred and wants to help him.

ASSESS

Based on your caregiver knowledge, if you were Jenny you might detect information similar to the following, with or without feedback from Fred.

Cognitive skill involved	Ability to start-sequence-stop tasks, ability to detect pain, ability to sense threat
Symptoms of decline	Inability to start-sequence-stop tasks, sense of threat, sense of urgency
Unmet need	BELONGING: Fred lacks social engagement PURPOSE: Fred lacks meaningful activities
Associated emotions	Anxious, lonely, bored, over-stimulated
Will	Will is exaggerated over power and ability

187

10 | APPLYING THE COMPASS RESPONSE TEMPLATE

Jenny has learned that pacing sometimes signals pain, not boredom. Fred's facial expression reinforces her guess that Fred is in physical distress. Jenny will ask a few yes-or-no questions to try to quickly assess what's happening so that any necessary medical response can be administered promptly.

"Is it a headache?" Is it an ear ache? Is your tooth bothering you again?"

If Jenny can't find a physical reason for Fred's pacing and distress, she will probe for an emotional trigger. *"I see the look on your face. Something's wrong. Can you tell me about it?"*

ATTEND

Jenny will attend to any physical need before addressing the emotions that have escalated. By talking with Fred she discovers that he is bored and lonely, talking to himself as he paces, unable to do anything on his own to change the situation.

Jenny suggests they go to the cafeteria and play cards. Fred still likes gin rummy, and they can enjoy fellowship there. Jenny hopes that other men Fred's age will also be there and that Jenny can introduce them to each other. If Fred made some friends he might have more activities and conversation during the day.

CONCLUSION

With myriad variables factoring in, each situation is different and it would be impossible to try to address each unique manifestation and escalation you may face now, and through the progression of dementia. But you don't need specific answers any longer. You now know how to problem solve your unique set of escalations as they present themselves.

Using the building blocks you've learned from this guide, you are ready to start applying the Compass Response Template and problem-solve for answers to your specific, individual situations. With dementia, there is no "perfect" care, but you can be confident that you are making possible the greatest number of "Good Nows" in the time that you have.

FIELD ASSIGNMENT:

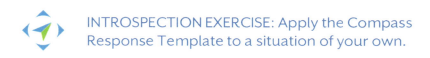 INTROSPECTION EXERCISE: Apply the Compass Response Template to a situation of your own.

Use the worksheet on the following page to apply the Compass Response Template to an escalated situation of your own that you would like to problem solve.

10 | APPLYING THE COMPASS RESPONSE TEMPLATE

COMPASS RESPONSE TEMPLATE WORKSHEET

ALIGN

COMPASS
3-2-1

APPROACH

Address
Request
Join
Validate

ASSESS

Physical
Environmental
Emotional

ATTEND

Take agency
Give agency
Transform

ANALYZE

Repeat
Revise
Replace

ANTICIPATE

Avert
Divert

10 | APPLYING THE COMPASS RESPONSE TEMPLATE

[i] James, O. (2008). *Contented dementia* (2nd ed.). Vermilion Pages. The suggestion in the text is inspired by a concept from UK dementia caregiving specialist Penny Garner, spelled out in this reference.

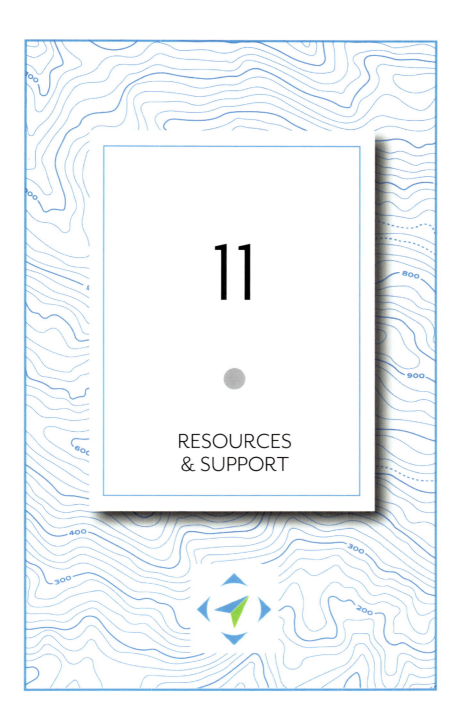

11

RESOURCES & SUPPORT

11 | RESOURCES & SUPPORT

> Eric restrains his anger in front of his teenage kids. He wants to be careful not to model a victim's attitude about putting his retirement plans on hold. He was going to sell the house and live the dream of writing his novel from a tiny cabin he built himself, tucked in a hollow high above the right bank of West Virginia's New River. His anger is natural, understandable. Still, he would like to show his boys his "better man" in difficult situations. So he saves the anger for his support group. Every member will support him in the absence of judgment and treat the conversation confidentially.

Are caregivers selfish to put themselves first? By definition, caregivers prioritize the needs of the person in their care. Their "default" mode becomes self-sacrifice. *Yet caregivers must have a whole self from which to give.*

We exhaust the fuel from our tank as we travel the caregiver's journey. We must replenish our fuel before the tank is empty. We must refill the tank completely to go the distance. Is it selfish to refuel our tank?

Is it selfish to replenish our bodies with nutrition, water, and rest? We don't think of these activities as selfish because they are necessary to our existence. But as we saw before, these are only some of our universal human needs.

It is not selfish to take care of your whole self properly. It is not selfish to try to fulfill all of your needs. Proper self-care optimizes well-being and makes possible the gift of your best self in caregiving. To compliment the self-care material detailed in Chapter Six, it's important to know of these additional resources to support you in caregiving.

RESOURCES

Current Research – The National Institute on Aging, at www.nia.nih.gov/health/alzheimers-disease-research-centers provides the most current science information through its national website and the 31 centers throughout the US.

Support Groups – Every caregiver should take advantage of the many benefits a support group offers. In a support group, all

194

11 | RESOURCES & SUPPORT

members are caregivers. Usually the group facilitators or leaders are or have been caregivers just like you. So everyone is very aware of what your current life is like.

Each member has an opportunity to share what's on their mind, whether it's a tactical question or an emotional issue. Members work together on the issues that arise.

Sometimes you'll get advice. Other times you'll give advice. What's said in the support group remains confidential. It is a safe culture that helps caregivers with knowledge, ideas, and emotional support. And without judgment. This time to bond with caregiving peers that are outside your family unit will be life changing.

Most groups meet for an hour. Some meet weekly, others monthly. Many now meet online. Both those I facilitate are now hosting online. It's amazing how the chemistry between members is not diminished even though these member bonds are not formed face to face. Find a support group that is convenient (so you'll go often).

Finding a support group can be achieved by asking the internet, your faith leader, medical practitioner, or local assisted living facility for a referral. Your local chapter of the Alzheimer's Association facilitates several support groups in your area as well. To find one near you, go to www.alz.org and search for your local chapter, then search for the support groups available in your area.

24/7 Toll-free Helpline – The Alzheimer's Association provides a dedicated helpline, crewed by people who are knowledgeable about dementia and can support you on a wide ranging list of dementia-related topics. I have had caregivers tell me that they've programmed the toll-free **800-272-3900** into their phones and use it often. It's nice to know there is always someone on the other end of the phone whether you need urgent advice or simply to further your knowledge.

Virtual Dementia Tour – The Virtual Dementia Tour® is a patented, scientifically proven method of building a greater understanding of dementia through the use of patented sensory tools and instruction. The Tour was created by P.K. Beville, PhD, an award-winning geriatric specialist and founder of Second Wind Dreams®. Proceeds from the sale of the Virtual Dementia Tour support the

11 | RESOURCES & SUPPORT

work of Second Wind Dreams, and international, nonprofit organization recognized as the first in the nation committed to changing the perception of aging through the fulfillment of dreams for elders. For more information about Second Wind Dreams visit www.secondwind.org.

Respite Care – Help is available when no one on your caregiving team is able to be with your loved one. Respite care makes it possible for you to go on vacation for much needed rejuvenation. There are numerous reasons why you might need a skilled professional outside your family to care for your loved one for a day or a weekend. Caregivers helping another family member move their residence, travelling to meet a new grandbaby for the first time, taking a much-needed vacation, or merely needing a Plan B when unforeseen circumstances affect the caregiving team schedule – these are just a few reasons to seek the support respite care can offer.

It may be that you hire someone to come to your home (preferable) or that you take your loved one to a facility offering respite care. There should be no shame in arranging respite care – professional or relative – when other options won't work. Respite care is not a cop-out.

Home Health Aides and Private Duty Nurses – Many families hire a professional caregiver for one-on-one support. A variety of scenarios are possible, from a few hours a week, to a few hours a day, to full day, or around the clock care. These caregivers can come to your home or an assisted living facility/memory care unit. Your medical team may be able to provide a referral and/or you can search online to find local providers, individuals, and companies.

One-on-One Mentoring – Caregivers may benefit from having an on-going relationship with a dementia mentor or coach. This is particularly helpful before and after diagnosis as well as when the person with dementia transitions from one stage to the next. These are the times when caregivers typically have the most questions and seek the most advice about dementia and the caregiving role.

This form of mentoring is usually experienced as hour-long, recurring sessions at first (three to ten sessions) while the caregiver

11 | RESOURCES & SUPPORT

learns the building blocks presented here and receives support in problem solving the individual scenarios they experience. Then, once the caregiver has found their bearings and is learning to navigate dementia, ad hoc or regular sessions create the on-going safety net to suit each caregiver.

If you are considering a dementia caregiver mentor, look for one who is skilled in dementia caregiving, adult education, and support group facilitation. Ask whether the mentor keeps relevant certifications active by undergoing annual performance reviews. It's important that a dementia caregiver mentor remain up to date on the medical as well as caregiving aspects of dementia.

Subscribe to The Dementia Caregiver Compass® Newsletter – Receive our free caregiver information monthly in your email Inbox. This newsletter is monthly. You may subscribe by going to www.newstreetcompass.com/newsletter

CONCLUSION

Equipped with the principles, tools, and resources presented in The Dementia Field Guide, you have everything you need to chart your course, navigate your way and problem-solve to remove obstacles your find along your path. Dementia caregiving is a journey like no other and there can be great joy in it.

Allow your curiosity to invite exploration into dementia and its particular presentation in your loved one. While many things may never be explained, you will identify patterns and find connections between your loved one's personality and identity and the symptoms he or she displays. With these connections your caregiving will become less about situations and more about relationships. Caregiving becomes easier, more productive, and more rewarding.

I wish you well on your journey.

11 | RESOURCES & SUPPORT

FIELD ASSIGNMENT:

 SOCIAL SUPPORT ACTIVITY: If you have not already done so, join a support group.

If you don't like the chemistry created by members of the first group you visit, find another group. Most support groups meet monthly. If you would like support more often, consider belonging to more than one group – there are no rules against it.

199

" Snatching the eternal out of the desperately fleeting is the great magic trick of human existence."

TENNESSEE WILLIAMS

202

ABOUT THE AUTHOR

Cloud Conrad based the principles, tools, and techniques presented in **The Dementia Field Guide** on research, industry best practices, personal caregiving experience, dementia-specific training, corporate training, and coaching training.

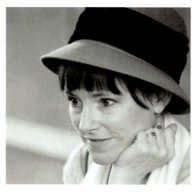

Conrad founded New Street Compass (https://*newstreetcompass.com*) to transform caregivers' sense of fear, frustration and failure into curiosity, creative problem solving, and confidence. Her work as a dementia caregiver trainer and mentor answers a call that she heard while caregiving for her father.

Conrad is a Certified Independent Caregiver Trainer (*Teepa Snow, Positive Approach to Care®*), Associate Certified Coach (*International Coach Federation*), Certified Trainer for the Virtual Dementia Tour® (Second Wind Dreams), Certified Creative Problem Solving Facilitator and Trainer (Creative Education Foundation), and Community Educator and Support Group Facilitator (*Alzheimer's Association*).

Conrad offers group classes, private classes, and one-on-one training/mentoring to professional and family dementia caregivers. She conducts the Virtual Dementia Tour® and trains others to facilitate the tour. She is a sought-after public speaker.

Conrad lives in Winder, Georgia. When not training and mentoring other dementia caregivers, she can be found gardening, hiking, kayaking, or making art in her studio.

204

APPENDICES

APPENDIX A:
WHEEL OF COGNITIVE FUNCTION   i

APPENDIX B
SIGNALS OF COGNITIVE DECLINE ASSESSMENT   iii

APPENDIX C:
CAREGIVER SELF-CARE & WELL-BEING ASSESSMENT   xv

APPENDIX A:

WHEEL OF COGNITIVE FUNCTION & DECLINE

The eight cognitive functions described in this book, and the way that they become impaired by dementia, have never before been organized in such a complete and concise manner, in any table or diagram, as "The Wheel of Cognitive Function and Decline".

Affectionately known as "The Wheel of Function" – or simply "The Wheel" – this diagram arrays the material on cognitive function concentrically, making it easier to remember the information. But this configuration also helps learners discover the connections which exist between skills, and their dysfunction, in various parts of the brain.

This pull-out guide complements the ideas and material presented in several chapters, tools, and field assignments as well as the Cognitive Skills Assessment in Appendix B.

It should be noted that the areas of the brain are not positioned in the diagram exactly as they are located in the skull. This is because the diagram cannot be presented three-dimensionally on paper.

The Wheel of Cognitive Function and Decline is original, copyrighted material conceived and created by Cloud Q. Conrad.

NOTES

SIGNALS OF COGNITIVE DECLINE ASSESSMENT

APPENDIX B:

SIGNALS OF COGNITIVE DECLINE ASSESSMENT

Many of the signs of cognitive decline can be attributed to normal aging. How would you know when cognitive health has declined to a point which deserves your concern? Ask yourself, to what extent are signals you may have noticed a loved one, impacting quality of life. This assessment is not to be construed as a medical diagnostic tool. It is an introspective exercise designed to help you gain insight through focused observation.

It may be helpful to save this assessment tool and review it in several months. Has anything changed? If so, what and how much? *You may make a blank copies of this assessment before you start for your personal use in order to monitor cognitive changes over time.*

Finally, this assessment can help to guide you to the words to express your concerns about what you're observing to your loved one. Then, if you think you should initiate a conversation about signals you've noticed, take the next step by reading and completing the exercises in Chapter Five, The Conversation.

SIGNALS OF COGNITIVE DECLINE ASSESSMENT

Determine which column heading most closely describes your observations for each gauge, and circle the corresponding number. Total the points for that signal.

Signal	Gauge	Does not apply	Seldom applies	Often applies	Usually applies	Score
VISUAL 1. Problems with object recognition or facial recognition	More than just "senior moments"	0	1	2	3	*Total all points below.*
	More than a temporary lapse	0	1	2	3	
	Unusual, not as it used to be	0	1	2	3	
2. Objects seem to hide in plain sight	More than just "senior moments"	0	1	2	3	*Total all points below.*
	More than a temporary lapse	0	1	2	3	
	Unusual, not as it used to be	0	1	2	3	
3. Startled by shadow or reflection or other eye trickery	More than just "senior moments"	0	1	2	3	*Total all points below.*
	More than a temporary lapse	0	1	2	3	
	Unusual, not as it used to be	0	1	2	3	

APPENDIX B

SIGNALS OF COGNITIVE DECLINE ASSESSMENT

VISUAL

Signal	Gauge					Score
4. Problems with depth perception (unrelated to new eyewear)	More than just "senior moments"	0	1	2	3	Total all points below.
	More than a temporary lapse	0	1	2	3	
	Unusual, not as it used to be	0	1	2	3	
5. Seeing things that are not actually there/hallucinations	More than just "senior moments"	0	1	2	3	Total all points below.
	More than a temporary lapse	0	1	2	3	
	Unusual, not as it used to be	0	1	2	3	

VISUAL SCORE: _____ of a possible 45.

Determine which column heading most closely describes your observations for each gauge, and circle the corresponding number. Total the points for that signal.

LINGUISTIC

Signal	Gauge	Does not apply	Seldom applies	Often applies	Usually applies	Score
6. Lapses in noun or pronoun recall/word loss	Unusual, not as it used to be	0	1	2	3	Total all points below.
	More than just "senior moments"	0	1	2	3	
	Interrupts the flow of daily living	0	1	2	3	

SIGNALS OF COGNITIVE DECLINE ASSESSMENT

		0	1	2	3	
LINGUISTIC	7. Apparent loss of thought mid-sentence					
	Unusual, not as it used to be	0	1	2	3	*Total all points below.*
	More than just "senior moments"	0	1	2	3	
	Interrupts the flow of daily living	0	1	2	3	
	8. Slower response times in conversation					
	Unusual, not as it used to be	0	1	2	3	*Total all points below.*
	More than just "senior moments"	0	1	2	3	
	Interrupts the flow of daily living	0	1	2	3	
	9. Social withdrawal, disengagement					
	Unusual, not as it used to be	0	1	2	3	*Total all points below.*
	More than just "senior moments"	0	1	2	3	
	Interrupts the flow of daily living	0	1	2	3	
	10. Repetitive phrases					
	Unusual, not as it used to be	0	1	2	3	*Total all points below.*
	More than just "senior moments"	0	1	2	3	
	Interrupts the flow of daily living	0	1	2	3	

APPENDIX B

SIGNALS OF COGNITIVE DECLINE ASSESSMENT

LINGUISTIC						
11. Misunderstandings	Unusual, not as it used to be	0	1	2	3	*Total all points below.*
	More than just "senior moments"	0	1	2	3	
	Interrupts the flow of daily living	0	1	2	3	
12. Unexpected outbursts	Unusual, not as it used to be	0	1	2	3	*Total all points below.*
	More than just "senior moments"	0	1	2	3	
	Interrupts the flow of daily living	0	1	2	3	
13. Inappropriate language	Unusual, not as it used to be	0	1	2	3	*Total all points below.*
	More than just "senior moments"	0	1	2	3	
	Interrupts the flow of daily living	0	1	2	3	

LINGUISTIC/RHYTHMIC/SONIC SCORE: _____ of a possible 72.

SIGNALS OF COGNITIVE DECLINE ASSESSMENT

Determine which column heading most closely describes your observations for each gauge, and circle the corresponding number. Total the points for that signal.

Signal	Gauge	Does not apply	Seldom applies	Often applies	Usually applies	Score
EXECUTIVE 14. Inappropriate behavior	Unusual, not as it used to be	0	1	2	3	*Total all points below.*
	More than just "senior moments"	0	1	2	3	
	Interrupts the flow of daily living	0	1	2	3	
15. Problems with planning	Unusual, not as it used to be	0	1	2	3	*Total all points below.*
	More than just "senior moments"	0	1	2	3	
	Interrupts the flow of daily living	0	1	2	3	
16. Problems making decisions/problems choosing	Unusual, not as it used to be	0	1	2	3	*Total all points below.*
	More than just "senior moments"	0	1	2	3	
	Interrupts the flow of daily living	0	1	2	3	

APPENDIX B

SIGNALS OF COGNITIVE DECLINE ASSESSMENT

EXECUTIVE

Signal	Gauge					Score
17. Trouble executing familiar tasks	Unusual, not as it used to be	0	1	2	3	*Total all points below.*
	More than just "senior moments"	0	1	2	3	
	Interrupts the flow of daily living	0	1	2	3	

EXECUTIVE SCORE: _____ of a possible 36.

Determine which column heading most closely describes your observations for each gauge, and circle the corresponding number. Total the points for that signal.

SENSORY - MOTOR

Signal	Gauge	Does not apply	Seldom applies	Often applies	Usually applies	Score
18. Noticeably slower movement	Unusual, not as it used to be	0	1	2	3	*Total all points below.*
	More than just "senior moments"	0	1	2	3	
	Interrupts the flow of daily living	0	1	2	3	
19. Inability to detect pain	Unusual, not as it used to be	0	1	2	3	*Total all points below.*
	More than just "senior moments"	0	1	2	3	
	Interrupts the flow of daily living	0	1	2	3	

SIGNALS OF COGNITIVE DECLINE ASSESSMENT

SENSORY - MOTOR					
20. Mumbling/poor enunciation	Unusual, not as it used to be	0	1	2	3	*Total all points below.*
	More than just "senior moments"	0	1	2	3	
	Interrupts the flow of daily living	0	1	2	3	
21. Handwriting increasingly difficult to read	Unusual, not as it used to be	0	1	2	3	*Total all points below.*
	More than just "senior moments"	0	1	2	3	
	Interrupts the flow of daily living	0	1	2	3	
22. Problems with fasteners	Unusual, not as it used to be	0	1	2	3	*Total all points below.*
	More than just "senior moments"	0	1	2	3	
	Interrupts the flow of daily living	0	1	2	3	

SENSORY – MOTOR SCORE: _____ of a possible 45.

APPENDIX B

SIGNALS OF COGNITIVE DECLINE ASSESSMENT

Determine which column heading most closely describes your observations for each gauge, and circle the corresponding number. Total the points for that signal.

Signal	Gauge	Does not apply	Seldom applies	Often applies	Usually applies	Score
23. Getting lost on familiar paths, routes	Unusual, not as it used to be	0	1	2	3	*Total all points below.*
	More than just "senior moments"	0	1	2	3	
	Interrupts the flow of daily living	0	1	2	3	
24. Missed appointments	Unusual, not as it used to be	0	1	2	3	*Total all points below.*
	More than just "senior moments"	0	1	2	3	
	Interrupts the flow of daily living	0	1	2	3	
25. Repetitive questions	Unusual, not as it used to be	0	1	2	3	*Total all points below.*
	More than just "senior moments"	0	1	2	3	
	Interrupts the flow of daily living	0	1	2	3	

NEW LEARNING

SIGNALS OF COGNITIVE DECLINE ASSESSMENT

LEARNING

Signal	Gauge					Score
26. Misplaced items	Unusual, not as it used to be	0	1	2	3	*Total all points below.*
	More than just "senior moments"	0	1	2	3	
	Interrupts the flow of daily living	0	1	2	3	

NEW LEARNING SCORE: _____ of a possible 36.

Determine which column heading most closely describes your observations for each gauge, and circle the corresponding number. Total the points for that signal.

Signal	Gauge	Does not apply	Seldom applies	Often applies	Usually applies	Score
27. Delusions, believing things that aren't true	Unusual, not as it used to be	0	1	2	3	*Total all points below.*
	More than just "senior moments"	0	1	2	3	
	Interrupts the flow of daily living	0	1	2	3	
28. Inability to "move on" to Plan B when things change	Unusual, not as it used to be	0	1	2	3	*Total all points below.*
	More than just "senior moments"	0	1	2	3	
	Interrupts the flow of daily living	0	1	2	3	

SURVIVAL

APPENDIX B

SIGNALS OF COGNITIVE DECLINE ASSESSMENT

SURVIVAL						
29. Heightened sense of urgency	Unusual, not as it used to be	0	1	2	3	Total all points below.
	More than just "senior moments"	0	1	2	3	
	Interrupts the flow of daily living	0	1	2	3	
30. Chronic, elevated anxiety	Unusual, not as it used to be	0	1	2	3	Total all points below.
	More than just "senior moments"	0	1	2	3	
	Interrupts the flow of daily living	0	1	2	3	

SURVIVAL SCORE: _____ of a possible 36.

SIGNALS OF COGNITIVE DECLINE ASSESSMENT

Record the scores from each cognitive function in the third column below. Compare these scores with the ranges provided in the columns to the right. Circle the corresponding score range. These response ranges should give you a sense of whether concern is warranted for any functional areas. This step should help to bring the bigger picture into focus. Just don't forget, a score of 2 or higher on any one of the 30 signals is a cause for concern.

Cognitive Function	# Signals Assessed	Function Score	Range and Response (lower values are better)		
			Probably Normal Aging	Concerns Exist, Monitor > Explore	Concerns Exist, Explore
Visual	5		0 – 15	16 – 30	31 - 45
Linguistic	8		0 – 24	25 – 48	49 - 72
Executive	4		0 – 12	13 – 24	25 - 36
Sensory-Motor	5		0 – 15	16 –30	31 - 45
New Learning	4		0 – 12	13 – 24	25 - 36
Survival	4		0 – 12	13 – 24	25 - 36
TOTALS	30		0 – 90	91 – 180	181 – 270

APPENDIX B

CAREGIVER SELF-CARE & WELL-BEING ASSESSMENT

APPENDIX C:

CAREGIVER SELF-CARE & WELL-BEING ASSESSMENT

The Caregiver Self-Care & Well-Being Assessment is designed to support caregivers in the pursuit of the fulfilment of their human needs, from the essentials to self-actualization.

For caregivers, attending to their own well-being is an on-going activity. One's state will naturally fluctuate over time but for caregivers, self-awareness is critical to detect and address decreases in well-being quickly.

Use this assessment to gain a baseline or "snap shot" of this moment in time. *You may make a blank copies of this assessment before you start for your personal use in order to monitor cognitive changes over time.*

First let's assess your current emotional state. Then we'll look at six aspects of self-care.

*For each aspect of well-being listed on the following pages, select the column header that most closely matches how frequently each of the six statements was **true for you over the last 14 days**, and circle the corresponding number in that row (ex: If you rarely ate several servings of fruit and vegetables daily, you would circle the "2" on the first row, under "SELDOM", and move to the second row to proceed accordingly).*

CAREGIVER SELF-CARE & WELL-BEING ASSESSMENT

Physical State	NEVER	SELDOM	OFTEN	USUALLY	ALWAYS
1. I ate a balanced diet including several servings of fresh fruit and vegetables every day.	1	2	3	4	5
2. I walked briskly, or did some other vigorous, heart healthy exercise daily.	1	2	3	4	5
3. I drank eight glasses of water each day.	1	2	3	4	5
4. I got eight hours of sleep each night.	1	2	3	4	5
5. I kept up with my prescribed medications.	1	2	3	4	5
6. I brushed my teeth and flossed daily.	1	2	3	4	5
Physical Subtotals *Subtotal your points from each column at right.*					
Add up the subtotals and record the total at far right.				Physical Scores Total	

(maximum of 30)

xvi

APPENDIX C

CAREGIVER SELF-CARE & WELL-BEING ASSESSMENT

Environmental State	(Respond based on your own home if not living with your loved one.)	NEVER	SELDOM	OFTEN	USUALLY	ALWAYS
7.	In my home, I was able to keep household clutter under control.	1	2	3	4	5
8.	I managed to keep up with the laundry, dishes, dusting and vacuuming.	1	2	3	4	5
9.	I had a comfortable place to relax when I had time.	1	2	3	4	5
10.	There was a place where I/we could welcome any visitors	1	2	3	4	5
11.	I had a place I could go outside, to unwind in the fresh air	1	2	3	4	5
12.	I took precautions to eliminate risk of injury in my home.	1	2	3	4	5
Environmental Subtotals	Subtotal your points from each column at right.					
	Environmental Scores Total					

Add up the subtotals and record the total at far right.

(maximum of 30)

CAREGIVER SELF-CARE & WELL-BEING ASSESSMENT

Cognitive State	NEVER	SELDOM	OFTEN	USUALLY	ALWAYS
13. I exercised my brain with crosswords, card games or board games of strategy.	1	2	3	4	5
14. I learned new information by studying a subject, language, instrument or hobby.	1	2	3	4	5
15. I was mentally "present" at work and could focus on the task at hand when I was working.	1	2	3	4	5
16. When things upset me, I could control my behavior regardless of my emotions.	1	2	3	4	5
17. The quality of my intellectual output was good.	1	2	3	4	5
18. When problems come up, I can think things through to find appropriate solutions.	1	2	3	4	5
Cognitive Subtotals *Subtotal your points from each column at right.*					
				Cognitive Scores Total	

Add up the subtotals and record the total at far right.

(maximum of 30)

CAREGIVER SELF-CARE & WELL-BEING ASSESSMENT

Social State	NEVER	SELDOM	OFTEN	USUALLY	ALWAYS
19. I could lean on a network of core people for support.	1	2	3	4	5
20. I was prepared with an answer if anyone asked, "What can I do to help?"	1	2	3	4	5
21. I was able to spend time with people I enjoy several times a week, whether on the phone or computer or in person.	1	2	3	4	5
22. I attended a support group for Alzheimer's and other dementia caregivers in the last four weeks		If NO, score 1. If YES, score 5			5
23. If a planned get together was canceled or rescheduled, I still connected and socialized in other ways.*	1	2	3	4	5
24. I took steps to create boundaries or otherwise distance myself from toxic people*	1	2	3	4	5
Social Subtotals					
Subtotal your points from each column at right.					
Add up the subtotals and record the total at far right.				Social Scores Total	

(maximum of 30)

If this did not apply in the last 2 weeks, score "3" for this question to create a neutral answer.

CAREGIVER SELF-CARE & WELL-BEING ASSESSMENT

Value State	NEVER	SELDOM	OFTEN	USUALLY	ALWAYS
25. Although I'm not perfect, I liked who I was and how I showed up.	1	2	3	4	5
26. I felt motivated by a sense of purpose.	1	2	3	4	5
27. I was able to contribute to the greater good in a meaningful way, outside of contributing to my family.	1	2	3	4	5
28. I felt welcome in a "community" of people who understand me.	1	2	3	4	5
29. I felt good that people needed my help.	1	2	3	4	5
30. My interests and ideas drove me to action.	1	2	3	4	5
Value Subtotals	*Subtotal your points from each column at right.*				
	Add up the subtotals and record the total at far right.			Value Scores Total	

(maximum of 30)

APPENDIX C

CAREGIVER SELF-CARE & WELL-BEING ASSESSMENT

Spiritual State	NEVER	SELDOM	OFTEN	USUALLY	ALWAYS
31. I was able to make enough time for myself.	1	2	3	4	5
32. I engaged in prayer, meditation or other contemplative activity.	1	2	3	4	5
33. I spent time exploring spiritual thought through readings, videos or discussion.	1	2	3	4	5
34. I was aware of my energy and recognized when it was time to rejuvenate.	1	2	3	4	5
35. I felt connected to something greater than myself.	1	2	3	4	5
36. I was able to see and savor beauty at least once a day.	1	2	3	4	5
Spiritual Subtotals	*Subtotal your points from each column at right.*				
	Add up the subtotals and record the total at far right.			Spiritual Scores Total	

(maximum of 30)

CAREGIVER SELF-CARE & WELL-BEING ASSESSMENT

Record your Aspect State scores (from the first section) in the corresponding row below.

Based on the Range and Response guidelines, is there an opportunity for improvement?

Aspect State	Number of questions	Subtotal Score	Range and Response (higher scores are better)		
			Address	Concern > Address	Balanced
Environmental	6		6 – 13	14 – 20	21 - 30
Physical	6		6 – 13	14 – 20	21 - 30
Spiritual	6		6 – 13	14 – 20	21 - 30
Cognitive	6		6 – 13	14 – 20	21 - 30
Social	6		6 – 13	14 – 20	21 - 30
Value	6		6 – 13	14 – 20	21 - 30
TOTAL	36		≤ 78	79 – 120	≥ 121

Are there aspects of your well-being that deserve attention? Chapter Six offers a guided work space to help you develop an action plan to address any aspect(s) and gauge your progress toward optimum well-being.

APPENDIX C

INDEX

3-2-1 *79, 147, 190*

Adrenaline *38, 134, 168*

Agitation *40, 134-5, 169, 173, 187*

Align *88, 117, 143, 145, 157, 159, 190*

Alzheimer's *7, 9, 18, 63, 71, 90, 113, 194, Appendix C*

Alzheimer's Association *9, 154, 195, 203*

Amygdalae *38-40, 133-135, Appendix A*

Analyze *152, 159, 190*

Anticipate *152, 159, 190*

Appendix A *17, 42, 90*

Appendix B *42, 48-9*

Appendix C *97-9*

Appointment Notes *124*

Approach *147, 160, 161, 163,166, 168, 172, 174, 177, 179, 182, 185, 187, 190*

Assess *147, 157, 159, 160, 162-3, 166, 169, 172, 175, 177, 179, 182, 185, 187, 190*

Assessment, Caregiver Self-Care *97-9, Appendix C*

Assessment, Signals of Cognitive Decline *42, 46, 48-51, Appendix B*

Attend *150, 161-2, 164, 167, 169, 173, 175, 178, 180, 183, 186, 188, 190*

Auditory processing *23-28*

Bad Nows *144*

Caregiver health risks *86*

Compass Response Template *145-54, 156-7, 159, 178, 188, 190*

Caregiving Team *115, 118, 122, 196*

Caveman *36, 38, 40*

Clumsiness *32, 34*

Cognitive Health Gauge *41-2, 47-8, 51-3, 80, Appendix B*

Cognitive stimulation *94-6*

Color recognition *19*

Communication of Emotions *136*

Communication shifts *135, 137-8*

Compensation *49, 173*

Completing sentences 24

Comprehension *24, 78, 135-6, 160, 167*

Conversation Template *75-9*

Covering *49*

Daily List *119-120, 123, 170*

Delusions *39, 50, 169, 171-4, Appendix A, Appendix B*

Dementia Caregiver Compass *58-67, 71, 73, 87-92, 156,*

Denial *72, 76, 78, 112, 114*

Depression *42, 46, 75-6, 86*

Depth perception *21, 50, Appendix A, Appendix B*

Diagnosis *9-10, 74-5, 112-4, 196*

Discomfort *147-8, 157, 160, 164, 176-7, 180, 183, 187*

Eccentric behavior *30, 90*

Elevated anxiety *38, 50, 160, 163, 172, Appendix A, Appendix B*

Escalation of Emotion *134-5, 156*

Emotions of Need *61-6, 150, 156*

Environmental triggers/aspects *99, 135, 147-9, 150-1, 173*

Episodic memories *37*

Escalated situations *12, 63, 131, 133-5, 138-9, 143, 145, 153, 156*

INDEX

Executive function 7, 29-31, 185, *Appendix A, Appendix B*
Exercise 93-6, 118, *Appendix C*
Facial recognition 19, 50, *Appendix A, Appendix B*
Family Plan 115-23
Fasteners, problems with 35, 50
Fatty diets 46, 93
Female caregivers 84-6
Fight or flight 38, 168
Fine motor skills 34-5, 93, 182
Frontotemporal Dementia 7, 29-30
Getting lost 36, 50, *Appendix A, Appendix B*
Good Nows 144, 188
Go-to phrases 184
Gross motor skills 34, *Appendix A*
Hallucinations 7, 50, 152, 171, 174-6 *Appendix A, Appendix B*
Hangry 133
Helen Keller *Foreword*
Helicopter 30
Hierarchy of Need 60, 61
Hippocampus 35-8, 40, 50, *Appendix A*
Home health aides, private duty nurses 196
Hot flashes 46
Human need fulfillment models 131-5
Illegible handwriting 34, 50, *Appendix A*
Immediate recall 36
Inappropriate acts/behavior 30, 50, 181, *Appendix A*
Inappropriate language 28, 50, 179-80, *Appendix A, Appendix B*

Infectious burden 46
Isolation 87, 92, 134-5, 148, 165, 180
Language/linguistic skills 23-8, 136-8, 167, 179, *Appendix A, Appendix B*
Left temporal lobe 23-5, *Appendix A*
Lewy Body Dementia 7
Life History 116, 121
Life Project 116, 121-3
Lifestyle Planning Template 96-7, 102-8
Limbic system 35, 40, *Appendix A*
Linguistic processing 23-25, *Appendix A*
Loneliness 92, 144, 149, 165, 166, 180
Lyme disease 46
Male caregivers 86
Mantras 89-90
Manual dexterity 34, 183
Mead, Margaret 85
Maslow, Abraham 60-1, 65, 131, 133
Mastery 132-4
Medial temporal lobe 35, 37, 40
Mehrabian, Albert 135-6
Memory 3, 7, 42, 46, 58, 73, 94, 150, 163, 166
Memory, lapse/loss/problems 7, 16, 46, 113, 157
Memory, and new learning 35-7, 47, 50, 94, 160, 162-3, 169 *Appendix A, Appendix B*
Memory, muscle 34
Memory, short term recall 136
Memory, working 16, 23, 149
Mentoring 196, 203
Mime 138

INDEX

Mini-Mental State Exam *113*

Misplaced objects *36, 50, Appendix A, Appendix B*

Missed appointments *36-7, 50, Appendix A, Appendix B*

Misunderstandings *6, 24, 27, 50, 138, Appendix A, Appendix B*

Motion blindness *20, Appendix A, Appendix B*

Mumbling *34-5, 50, Appendix A, Appendix B*

National Institute on Aging *194*

Needs *60-3, 65-6, 87, 89, 91-2, 97, 116, 131, 133, 137-9, 140, 143, 147, 150, 156, 159, 194, Appendix C*

Needs, unmet/unfulfilled *131, 133-4, 137-9, 143, 147*

Needs, and escalations *39, 62-3, 134, 138-9, 143, 145, 147, 174, 180-2,*

Newsletter, electronic *197*

Non-verbal cues *136-8, 151*

Nutrition *92-3, 96, 194*

Object recognition *19, 50, Appendix A, Appendix B*

Occipital lobe *19, 21*

Occupational hazards *86*

Odor *40*

Olfactory gland *33, 40*

Pain *33, 50, 143, 147-9, 157, 160, 175-9, 187-8, Appendix A, Appendix B*

Perfect, perfection *152-3, 188, Appendix C*

Peripheral vision, field of vision *20-1, 178, 182, Appendix A, Appendix B*

Personal Fact Sheet *116, 121, 123, 127, 181*

Person-centered care *117, 130*

Plan B *39, 50, 196, Appendix A, Appendix B*

Positron Emission Tomography (PET) *17-8, 21, 113*

Pre-frontal cortex, pre-frontal lobe *29, 183, 184, Appendix A*

Prescription drugs *46, 114*

Proprioception, proprioceptors *32-3*

Radar graph *98-101, 102-8*

Reflections *176*

Reminiscing *122, 164, 166-7*

Repetitive actions *186-7*

Repetitive questions *36-7, 50, 152, 159-65, Appendix A, Appendix B*

Respite care *196*

Rhythmic processing *26-8, Appendix A, Appendix B*

Right temporal lobe *23-4, 26-8, 136, 173, 180, 184, Appendix A*

Risk *185*

Risk, factors *7-9, 48*

Risk, caregiver *86, 101*

Routine *116, 118, 121, 174*

Rummaging *130, 185-6*

Sacrifice *86, 88, 194*

Self-control *29-30, 179, Appendix A*

Self-Care *12, 86-8, 91-9, 101, 116, 194, Appendix C*

Self-Care, Action Plan *86, 99-108, Appendix C*

Self-care, maintenance *102-8*

Self-preservation *35-40, 85*

Self-worth *60, 87-8, 170*

Sensory processing *31-3, 195*

Sequencing tasks *29, 183-4, Appendix A, Appendix B*

INDEX

Set Test *113*

Seven Minute Screen *113*

Shadows *20, 176, Appendix A, Appendix B*

Shuffling *34*

Signals of cognitive decline *16-42*

Signals of Cognitive Decline Inventory *49-51*

Sleep *95-7, Appendix C*

Slowed movement *34, 50, Appendix A, Appendix B*

Social chit chat *26-7, 138, 167, 180*

Social engagement *94-5, 97, 168, 183-4, 187*

Social withdrawal *24, 50, Appendix A, Appendix B*

Sonic processing *26-8, 136, Appendix A, Appendix B*

Spatial relationships *23-4, 32, 34*

Speech production *136-7*

Spiritual time, spirituality *95, 97, 99, Appendix C*

Support Group *Foreword, 91-2, 97, 194-5, 197-8, 203, Appendix C*

Symptoms *7, 10-12, 42, 62-3, 66, 75-6, 90, 114, 130, 133, 135, 139, 145, 146, 156, 159, 197, Appendix A, Appendix B*

Symptom-related behaviors *63, 182*

Tay and Dienier research *133*

Thyroid problems *46*

Toll-free helpline *195*

Tracking Cognitive Health Schedule *49*

Too's *149*

Unexpected outbursts *33, 50*

Unresolved issues *90*

US Census *9*

Vascular Dementia *7*

Verbal cues *136-8, 151*

Verbal outbursts *178-81, Appendix A, Appendix B*

Violent outbursts *176-8, Appendix A, Appendix B*

Visual cues *19, 136-8*

Visual processing *19-22, 136-8, 175-6, 178, Appendix A, Appendix B*

Vocabulary *23, 25, 28, 136, 149*

Voice modulation *138*

Wandering *168, 171*

Water *95-6, Appendix C*

Wayfinding *36, 168, Appendix A, Appendix B*

Well-being *Foreword, 7, 8, 12, 59, 76, 86-8, 91-2, 97-9, 101-8, 133, 135, 142-3, 150, 159, 164, 172, 194, Appendix C*

Well-being gauge *98-100, Appendix C*

Wheel of Cognitive Function *17, 42, 90, 139, Appendix A*

Wildebeests *36, 38*

Will, power, ability *62-3, 66, 131-5, 138, 150, 156-7, 161, 164-5, 167, 169, 175, 178, 180, 183, 186, 188*

Word loss *23-4, 50, Appendix A, Appendix B*

ORDER ADDITICNAL COPIES OF THE DEMENTIA FIELD GUIDE

You may purchase additional copies of this book from www.dementiafieldguide.com. Or, you may purchase offline with a valid check, printed by an FDIC banking institution, that includes your address and phone number. Complete this form and return it to the address below, along with your check made **payable to Cloud Conrad** in the total amount due.

⬇ BILLING INFO　　　　　　　⬇ SHIP TO

_____

_____

_____

_____

 Your email (*required*)
_____
 Your daytime phone (*required*)
_____

Write the total number of books you'll order in the box with the ➔ symbol. Multiple that number by the **total cost** of each book and write that total in the blue box with the **$**.

Item	Cost (each)	QUANTITY/TOTAL	
The Dementia Field Guide	$32.50	➔	
Shipping	$ 3.50	X	$36.00 =
TOTAL COST	**$36.00**	$	

Mail this form and your check, in the above amount, to:

Cloud Conrad
91 W. New Street,
Winder, GA 30680

For orders of five or more books, price inquiries can be initiated using this form, mailed to the address above.